your best body

Michelle Bridges has worked in the fitness industry for over twenty years as a professional trainer and group fitness instructor. Her role in Channel Ten's hit reality show *The Biggest Loser* combined with her highly successful online exercise and mindset program, the 12 Week Body Transformation, has connected her with hundreds of thousands of Australians, making her this country's most recognised and influential fitness personality. *Your Best Body* is her seventh book. Her previous books – *Crunch Time, Crunch Time Cookbook, Losing the Last 5 Kilos, 5 Minutes a Day, The No Excuses Cookbook* and *Everyday Weight Loss* – are all bestsellers.

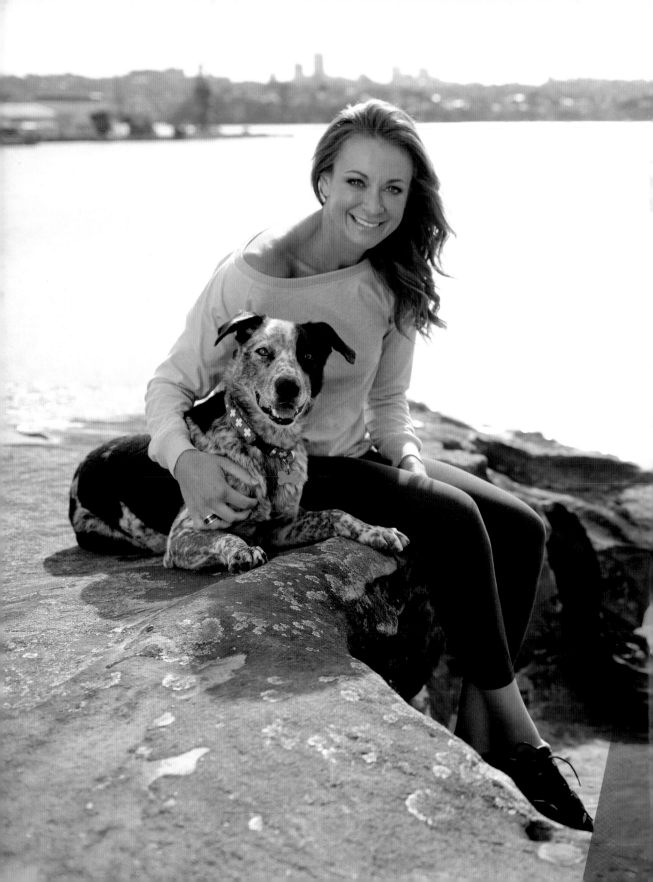

your best body

BEST *thinking*
BEST *training*
BEST *eating*

Get the results you want

michelle bridges

VIKING
an imprint of
PENGUIN BOOKS

To my long-term mate and personal trainer Joey Sheather
who got me in rip-roaring shape for 'train the trainer'
on *The Biggest Loser.* We kicked arse mate! Cheers!

Joey, this book is dedicated to you and your family. xxx

VIKING

Published by the Penguin Group
Penguin Group (Australia)
707 Collins Street, Melbourne, Victoria 3008, Australia
(a division of Pearson Australia Group Pty Ltd)
Penguin Group (USA) Inc.
375 Hudson Street, New York, New York 10014, USA
Penguin Group (Canada)
90 Eglinton Avenue East, Suite 700, Toronto, Canada ON M4P 2Y3
(a division of Pearson Penguin Canada Inc.)
Penguin Books Ltd
80 Strand, London WC2R 0RL England
Penguin Ireland
25 St Stephen's Green, Dublin 2, Ireland
(a division of Penguin Books Ltd)
Penguin Books India Pvt Ltd
11 Community Centre, Panchsheel Park, New Delhi – 110 017, India
Penguin Group (NZ)
67 Apollo Drive, Rosedale, North Shore 0632, New Zealand
(a division of Pearson New Zealand Ltd)
Penguin Books (South Africa) (Pty) Ltd
Rosebank Office Park, Block D, 181 Jan Smuts Avenue, Parktown North, Johannesburg, 2196, South Africa
Penguin (Beijing) Ltd
7F, Tower B, Jiaming Center, 27 East Third Ring Road North, Chaoyang District, Beijing 100020, China

Penguin Books Ltd, Registered Offices: 80 Strand, London, WC2R 0RL, England

First published by Penguin Group (Australia), 2013

10 9 8 7 6 5 4 3 2 1

Text copyright © Michelle Bridges 2013
Photographs copyright © Nick Wilson
Food photography copyright © Julie Renouf

Cover and text design by Adam Laszczuk © Penguin Group (Australia)
Cover and author photographs by Nick Wilson
Food photography by Julie Renouf, home economy by Caroline Jones, food styling by Georgia Young
Food consultant Lucy Nunes
Typeset in Gotham by Adam Laszczuk, Penguin Group (Australia)
Colour reproduction by Splitting Image, Clayton, Victoria
Printed and bound in China by South China Printing Co Ltd

National Library of Australia
Cataloguing-in-Publication data:

Bridges, Michelle.
Your best body / Michelle Bridges.
ISBN: 9780670076383 (pbk.)
Exercise. Health. Weight loss.
613.7

penguin.com.au

CONTENTS

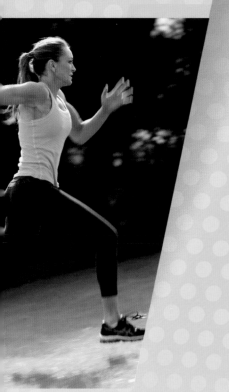

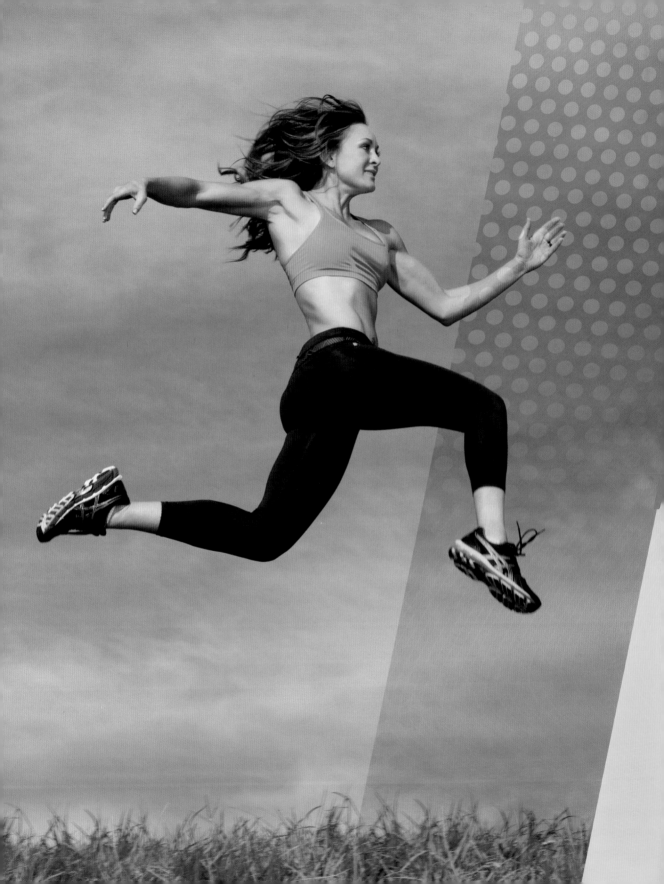

INTRODUCTION

'The human body is the universe in miniature. That which cannot be found in the body, is not to be found in the universe. Hence the philosopher's formula, that the universe within reflects the universe without. It follows therefore, that if our knowledge of our own body could be perfect we would know the universe.' - **MAHATMA GANDHI**

On the face of it my life's work appears to be about weight loss and helping people regain control of their weight through diet and exercise. The last book I wrote that featured exercise and menu plans was *Losing the Last Five Kilos*, and it offered a four-week program that promised just that – the tools to shake off the last few stubborn kilos and get people to their ideal weight.

I was overwhelmed by the success stories that people have shared with me having followed the training regimes and meal plans in those pages.

Some of them have gone on to lose seven, ten or 12 kilos, renewing their lives and reinvigorating their zest for living. I feel truly humbled to have been a catalyst in that process.

But weight loss isn't the whole story. My mission isn't to slim down Australia or the United Kingdom or anywhere else on the planet. Nor is it to have larders all over the world brimming with nutritious wholefood.

My mission is to re-empower people. To help people to take back control of their lives, and in doing so to control their outcomes. And for those people to pass it forward to their children, their families and their friends.

Modern lifestyles have a way of draining our power and self-responsibility. By providing things to make our everyday lives easier, today's world has quietly shifted our attention away from looking after ourselves to looking after our careers, our mortgages and our social lives.

It's as if we don't have the time to devote to the fundamental tenets of our existence – our bodies, our minds, our spirits. These basic elements have been overshadowed by new urgencies, the urgencies of twenty-first century living.

We now seem to spend so much time fretting about how our superannuation is looking and whether or not we'll have that marketing plan ready for the sales conference. If we'll be home in time from work to put the bins out, or how we'll get by if the home-loan interest rates go up by half a percentage point.

It's not that there's anything wrong with that. All of these things have a place in our lives; they all need our attention. But it's when the truly important things in our world have to take a back seat because we simply don't have the time, the energy or the focus to look after them and give them the attention they need - that's when our lives can become distorted.

This shift has also been detrimental to our inner strength. As a community, we've gone soft.

What this book is about is the most important thing in this world, in your world. **The thing that underpins everything**, that is the base on which everything else – from your relationship with your children to your effectiveness in your job – depends. It's about **your body**.

I know that might sound superficial. We live in an age in which there are so many competing pressures on our time and attention that focusing on your body rather than the mortgage or the kids may seem indulgent or unimportant. But it is essential.

I'm inviting you not to put your kids or your mortgage first. I'm inviting you to put you and your health first. Because by being a fitter, healthier, happier person you will be a better parent, employer, grandparent. It's no coincidence that during an aeroplane safety demonstration you're asked to put on your own oxygen mask first before helping others.

That is because it all starts and ends with you, and you alone. **You will always be able to look after others better when you have taken the trouble to look after yourself.** How can you look after your kids if you're chronically unwell yourself? Or enjoy your grandchildren if you're constantly in and out of hospital? Or support your family if you're too sick to work?

This isn't about going to the gym instead of working an hour overtime to help with a mortgage payment, or buying the latest overpriced organic berry instead of buying schoolbooks. It's about consistently investing in your physical self.

Of course, this book will give you all the tools you need to build **a slammin' set of shoulders, a tight midsection and a shapely pair of legs**. Follow the eating and exercise programs and you'll soon notice the difference, as will those around you.

But ultimately it's about being the best version of you.

Now, this book doesn't promise a transformation from a 'pear' to a spot on the runway at the next Victoria's Secret lingerie launch, or an express route to a berth on the Olympic swim team. *Your Best Body* promises just what it says – the best body you can get. Not the most muscular body, or the best for tackling marathons. It promises the most functional, lean, effective body for your life. It promises a body that is flexible and agile, but strong and powerful. It's about a body that is efficient and enduring. It gives you the opportunity to make the absolute most out of the body that you have been blessed with. Something always strikes me when I go through the process of writing a book, and the more I researched this one, going back over the chapters, examining and questioning why certain ideas and philosophies have turned up for me at this point in time, the more I saw one common thread running throughout. And the common thread is that this book, and indeed the whole principle of achieving your best body, isn't really about exercises and circuits, nor is it about superfoods or menu plans.

It's about **acceptance**.

The amazing collection of molecules and particles that make up your body is uniquely yours, and you have the opportunity to look after it, nourish it and honour it any way you choose. That, in itself, is a gift. It's a gift that we often take for granted though, and we can easily forget that it should be handled carefully and from a place of love.

Because *loving* your body – no matter what it looks like – is the first step to looking after it and cultivating it to be the very best that it can be. **With love comes respect, and with respect comes acknowledgement.** Acknowledging your body for what it is – how it looks, what it can and can't do – frees you up to find a place of acceptance.

Accepting the way we are is crucial to getting ourselves in the right mental state to find happiness in our physical selves and move forward positively. Sure, you can make changes to your body with diet and exercise. Your body will do exactly what you tell it to do, so changing it is always a possibility. But doing the work to change your mental state, the way that you think, can be an even bigger challenge.

This book will give you the tools to do this work, to change the way that you think and the way you perceive things. These tools will work hand in hand with the exercise programs and recipes, and will get you on the road not only to a healthy body, but to a **good mental state and a positive attitude to life** as well.

Recent research has confirmed what many of us have long suspected: that there is a direct relationship between the way we think – our moods, our cognitive powers – and what we eat and how we exercise.

Exercise more, and your heart and lungs will become stronger and more effective. Eat better, and all the millions of metabolic processes that take place every day will be more efficient, and your body will respond by staying alive longer and resisting disease better. But these changes can also influence the power of your brain and your attitude to life.

Most of us at some stage have been unhappy with our bodies. Maybe we think we're not tall enough or that our body is the wrong shape. But it's pointless to bitch about what you've been given. Some things you can change, some things can't, but at the end of the day, it's your body. No one else's; yours alone. And it's perfect. It isn't less perfect because it's twenty kilos overweight or because it's muscles aren't very strong. Those things are simply the result of the food and exercise messages it's been given over the years; it is just doing as it's told.

Happily, **your body is amazingly responsive** if you change those messages. Following the ideas in this book will make your body the most efficient, enduring, disease-free collection of cells that it can possibly be.

Will it look any different? Yep.

Will it reward you by offering more energy, more vitality, more longevity? You better believe it!

Will it improve your happiness and sense of wellbeing? Hell, yeah!

Will it allow you to enjoy your life to its fullest? No doubt about it.

The 'Your' in the title of this book is significant – you should be nourishing and exercising your body for you, and you alone. Not for your kids, or to keep your partner happy.

I often hear *The Biggest Loser* contestants standing on the scales telling the world that they need to lose weight and they're 'doing it for my kids' or 'for my husband'. Why would you make a commitment to look after yourself because somebody else wants you to, just to make *them* happy? Other people's happiness is their responsibility, not yours, so do it for you.

The 'Best' in the title refers to your body being the best version that it can be. It's not different – taller, wider, lighter – necessarily. It's still the same body, your body, but it's the best version of it.

The 'Body', importantly, means your whole body. It's your best skin, best brain, best liver. It's your best immune system and blood sugar levels. It's your best heart and digestive tract. The best you can make it by following a healthy nutritious diet and exercising regularly.

I'm going to give you all the tools you need to think right, train right and eat right – so you can **fulfil your potential** and get your best body.

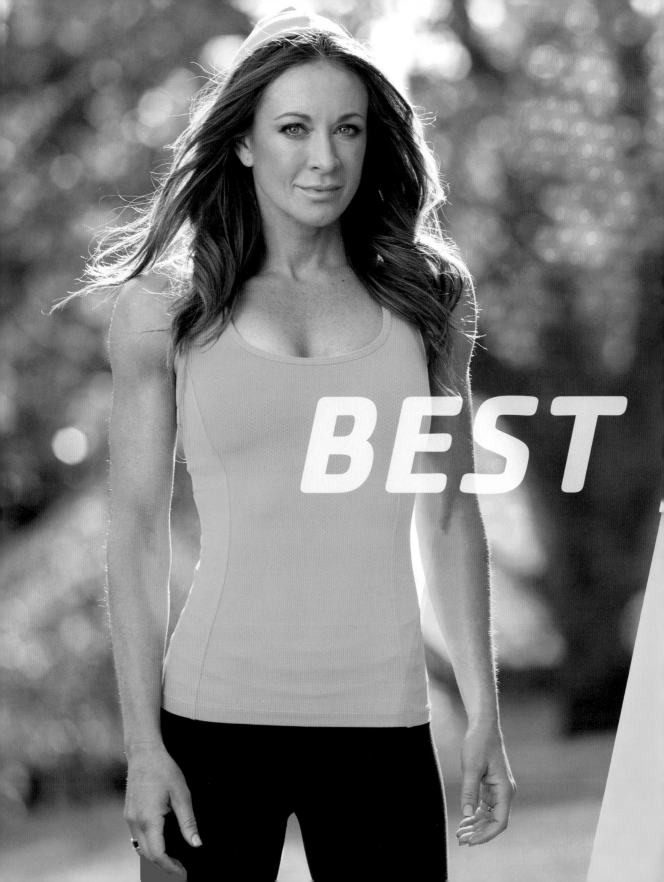

thinking

The first step towards realising the best version of yourself is understanding who you are, accepting that person and moving forward from a place of love and self-respect. Ditching negative traits such as comparisons with others will free you up to develop your own unique self into its best expression.

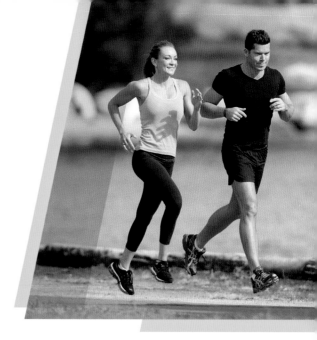

GETTING YOUR HEAD RIGHT

THE COMPARISON TRAP

Comparing ourselves to others is one of the most destructive things we can do to ourselves. Yet we all do it, particularly us girls. Before getting into all the emotional stuff around this subject, it's worth reminding ourselves *why* we are all different, and why **it's important that we aren't all the same**.

In order for a species to survive it needs to protect itself from disease, and changes in the environment and things like food availability. If we were all absolutely identical – same genetic make-up, same size, same allergies, same immune systems – a single environmental change or disease could wipe the species out, because our identical make-up wouldn't allow for differences that would offer protection to some members of the tribe.

This is why conservationists get so concerned when the number of a particular species of wild animal falls to very low levels. We could simplistically assume that as long as there are two of them, a male and a female, a species can survive because it can reproduce. But unless there are thousands of healthy individuals there simply isn't sufficient bio-individuality left in the group to cope with fluctuations that are part of everyday existence on the planet.

So, far from wanting to be like others, at an anthropological level we should be celebrating that we aren't. Our differences are the reason we're here.

There's no point in comparing ourselves with others because we are all individuals, and that's the way we should be. If you know someone who lost 3 kilos in three weeks by following this book, it doesn't mean that you will. If you've always wanted catwalk legs, but you were born with legs like a rugby league player, don't fight it; celebrate it.

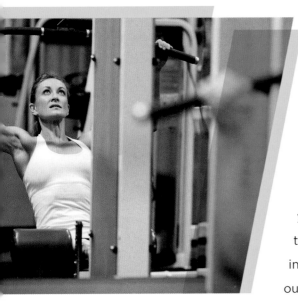

Magazine and advertising images have almost single-handedly messed up our collective heads when it comes to how we see ourselves in the context of others. I reckon I'm in a pretty good position to make a call on this, because in my line of work I regularly have to stand in front of a camera, usually wearing an outfit that looks like it's made of cling film.

And I'm here to tell you that it isn't something you can walk off the street and do. I routinely have to give myself a few weeks of intense preparation including clinical eating, excruciating gym workouts, regular sleep, gallons of spring water and, oh, did I mention excruciating gym workouts?

Which is all fine until we start to see these magazine physiques as normal everyday bodies, and use them as a reference point for how we should look. They're not how the vast majority of us look; in fact, frequently they're not even *real* having undergone some diligent photoshopping.

Comparing our physical selves with others is not just bad; it's disastrous. There can never be a good outcome. There will always be someone who is slimmer, more athletic, or more photoshopped.

Sometimes us girls get caught in the comparison trap when we're introduced to another girl. You know what I mean, the old quick-glance-up-and-down then 'The Appraisal', 'She's fatter than me, so that's OK', or 'Damn!

> *It is in comparisons that we tend to find fault with ourselves. Avoiding comparisons is the first step to a more positive outlook.*

I look older than her!' It's destructive and silly. If you find yourself doing it, pull yourself up and make a promise that next time you are consciously *not* going to do it. Trust me – it makes life a lot easier.

INSPIRATION AND ASPIRATION

Not comparing yourself with others doesn't mean that you can't be inspired by other people, inspired by what they have achieved or how they look. **Inspiration is really important as it is the precursor to thoughts, and thoughts lead to action.**

But there's a risk of confusing *inspiration* with *aspiration*. It's one thing to be inspired by others, but it's a completely different thing to aspire to be like them. Aspiration can never be truly fulfilled – we can't really be like other people – so inevitably we will be disappointed. Aspiration can be destructive.

Aspiration to look a certain way needs to be tempered with a big steaming cup of reality with two heaped teaspoons of acceptance. When you hear yourself saying 'I want to look like him/her', the alarm bells should start ringing. For most of us, that is something we will never achieve. But don't let that stand in the way of pursuing a healthy lifestyle, training hard and eating well, because your results will always be spectacular, and getting you towards the best version of *you.*

ACCEPTANCE

There is great **power in acceptance**. Once we take that step – *accepting* our bodies – we move past frustration and feelings of helplessness with ourselves to the opposite end of the emotional spectrum, to a place of empowerment. Wrestling with stuff that you can't change is exhausting. **Letting go of things that you can't change is liberating.**

Even if you can't change something, changing the way you think about it can give you a fresh perspective and enable you to move forward.

Try it. Think of something that really bugs you but you know, deep down, there's nothing you can do to change. Maybe it's that you have pale skin, or that your sister married someone you don't particularly like. Then simply cut it loose. Stop giving it the oxygen it needs to exist. It'll still be there, but it can no longer irritate you because you've taken away what it needs to do so. *You* gave it the power to get under your skin, and *you* can take that power back.

I recommend that when you think about yourself, you **put your health firmly into the equation over and above your appearance.** So every time you ask yourself 'How do I look?', also ask 'How healthy am I? What have I eaten, and what exercise have I done? What are the choices that I've made that support my health? And what choices will I make for the rest of today, and tomorrow?'

A STORY ABOUT ACCEPTANCE

There once was a man who was hunting deer in New Zealand. It was late autumn, and he was camped deep in the forests of the North Island. He took his hunting seriously, and was respectful of his quarry.

While making his way through the dense forest he noticed deer tracks in the mud of a shady clearing. The tracks were fresh, and he knew from the pattern of hoof prints that it was an area that was regularly visited by the animals. He made a note of the location and decided to go back there closer to dusk.

The following afternoon he set off to go back to the clearing. It was cold and the wind was blowing a few flakes of icy sleet across the narrow overgrown track that wound it's way to within four or five hundred metres of the clearing.

Although the shadowy glade was only around half a kilometre from the track, like most of the New Zealand bush the vegetation was dense, and it was a full hour's struggle through the ferns and vines that grew almost on top of each other to get there.

The New Zealand bush is notoriously unfriendly. Fallen trees, vines hanging low, bristling with savage hooks, grasses that can cut like paper. The canopy above is dense, allowing only the occasional glimpse of sunlight, and the hunter recalled the numerous volunteer searches for fellow hunters he had participated in over the years, some of which were not successful.

Arriving at the clearing he settled quietly and waited, his rifle loaded, cocked and ready. He didn't have to wait long. He could hear a deer working through the undergrowth, and he could almost smell the animal. A brief glimpse of antlers, a hint of the sheer size of the stag behind layers of vegetation, but not enough for a clear shot. So he waited. And waited.

He realised that the light would soon fade, and that time was working against him. He knew he was only a heartbeat away from his prize and that any second the beast could burst through the undergrowth into the clearing, breath steaming and standing proud.

But as night started to draw in the hunter sensed that the balance of risk was starting to tip away from the deer towards himself. It was time to move, and move quickly. He checked his compass and made his way into the maze of vines and grasses.

Suddenly, the light was all but gone. The dense canopy of the towering rata and rimu trees shut out the last of the sunlight in what seemed like a few brief moments. The hunter felt a twinge of panic as he realised that he had stayed too late, and that unless he could make it to the track very soon he faced an uncertain evening.

In his haste he made mistakes. With hook grass hacking at his legs, he stumbled into a thick growth of the bush lawyer vine and was instantly covered in its tentacles, ripping at him and frustrating all his efforts to release himself.

But it got worse – his compass was telling him that he had been walking in the opposite direction to the track. In his panic, he had been making his way deeper into the forest.

His immediate response was one of ego – 'How can that be? I'm experienced in the bush; there's no way I could get my direction that wrong! This compass isn't working . . .'

But the compass was working. In his growing panic he had totally lost his bearings. The twinge of fear became a deluge, as he turned round and thrashed his way through the undergrowth, now in almost total darkness.

Then something happened. He stopped, panting – his forehead slick with sweat or blood – stepped back and took stock. He was surrounded by the silence of the forest, and rather than fighting its quietness and solitude, he allowed himself to be immersed in it and started to take stock.

'Hang on. What's the worst that can happen here?'

His logical thoughts had been smothered by desperation, a desperation that wasn't needed. This was a time for clear thinking.

'So, here's how it is,' he told himself. 'I get to spend a night in the bush. Not my first choice, but there's not much I can do about it. Yes, it's cold, but I've got water and a compass, and when it's light, I can find the track and walk out of here.'

The sense of relief the hunter felt was almost overwhelming. Far from panicking, he was now almost jubilant. By accepting the way things were he had totally liberated himself. He was no longer trapped in the forest; he was *free* in the forest. He had accepted his situation without fear or blame.

The lesson he had learned was one that he would carry with him for the rest of his life, and he would go on to pass it to his children and others.

The next day, after a cold and unsettled night, he woke up and walked out of the forest, as he knew he would.

This is a true story. It happened near Lake Okataina in New Zealand's North Island in 1979. I know it's true because the hunter is my husband.

Acceptance involves maturely, thoughtfully and consciously accepting who and where you are at a particular moment in time. **Our bodies are perfect because they respond perfectly to what we tell them to do.** Acceptance is intrinsically linked to understanding this 'perfect body' concept.

When you exercise your body regularly and feed it well, it will respond perfectly and stay trim and healthy. If you feed it junk food and lead a sedentary lifestyle, it will respond accordingly by storing fat and losing lean muscle mass. It is the perfect piece of machinery. Nothing on this planet comes close!

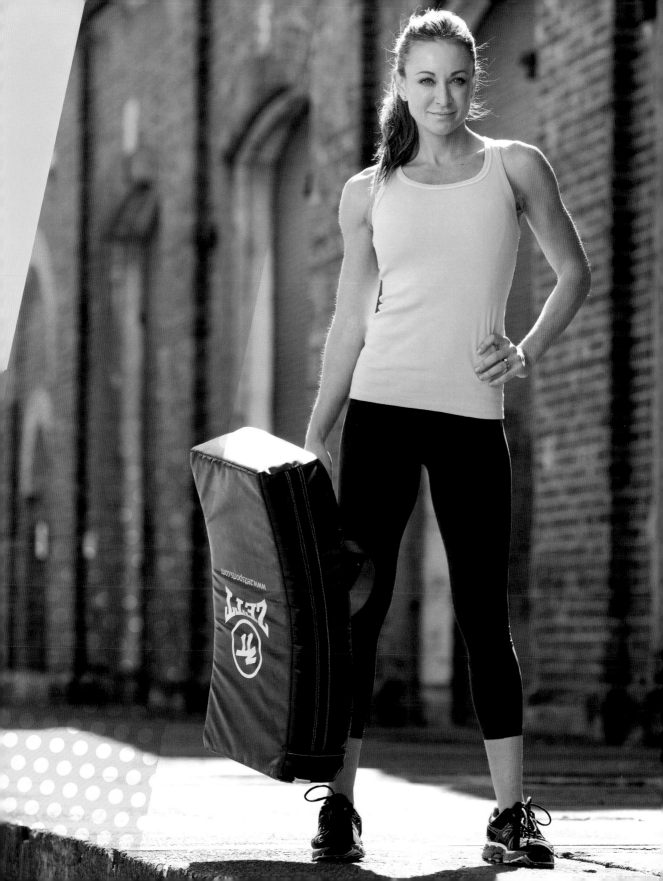

In my first book, *Crunch Time,* I spoke about how when we resist things in our lives, rather than making them go away, they persist. The notion of acceptance is also inextricably linked to the 'What you resist persists' principle, which asks you to accept that you are overweight, accept that you eat too much, accept that you don't like to exercise, and accept that you make excuses about all of this. No blame, no beat-ups, no guilt. Just be with it and accept responsibility for it.

'Pain is inevitable, suffering is optional' – **BUDDHA**

Own that you choose to be who you are today. Because it is only when you own who you are today that can you **take responsibility** for it. When you understand that you and you alone are responsible, you can then be equally responsible to effect change. It's only when you take total ownership of the way you are that you can move forward.

In my husband's story, had he not accepted his situation, he would have pressed on, panicked and made the situation far worse than it already was.

Acceptance is incredibly liberating, but we all struggle to incorporate it into our lives. I regularly hear statements from people along the lines of, 'Oh, Michelle, I just need to lose this middle-age spread! I feel so old and frumpy. Look at this stomach! It's dreadful!' or 'I hate myself! I can't fit into any of my clothes and I'm embarrassed to go out!'

Somewhere back in our past we've decided that if we berate ourselves enough, judge ourselves unfavourably enough, malign ourselves enough, belittle ourselves enough, then that will be the rocket up our backsides to get us moving and make a change.

How can making us feel bad about ourselves be the catalyst for lifelong change? How can self-criticism, even self-loathing, support us to be the best version of ourselves? Does it work? Maybe it temporarily shifts our thinking for a couple of days, but then we always go back to our old ways because our motivation *hasn't come from a place of love.*

> *Surround yourself with positivity and shut off the negative self–talk. Stay focused on your goals and know that beating yourself up is not the way to get motivated.*

The end result in the 'acceptance' cycle is love of self. **Loving ourselves for who we are** is critical to how we feel about ourselves, which in turn affects our relationships with others. Belittling ourselves with negative self-talk isn't, and never will be, about love of self. It's actually self-fulfilling because the inevitable sense of failure that follows is far more damaging than being overweight will ever be!

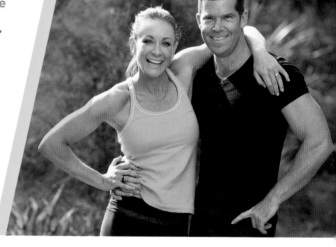

Sometimes we misguidedly use negative self-talk to motivate ourselves. But this motivation can only be temporary, because if we berate ourselves enough we actually start to *believe* the negative self-talk. What started as our perception can quickly become our reality.

But how can accepting my problems and issues motivate me to change them? If I accept them, then why would I bother to change them? Right?

Well, **acceptance is the conduit to change**. All of the facets of your life – health, fitness, career, relationships, whatever – are available for change once you accept them for what they are. It is the first step in moving forward.

'When you begin to accept yourself the way you are right now, you begin a new life with new possibilities that did not exist before because you were so caught up in the struggle against reality that that was all you could do'

– MANDY EVANS

TRAVELLING FREE: How to recover from the past by changing your beliefs

SELF-SUPPORT /

Something else changes when you accept yourself the way you are – you become self-supporting. You have the quiet confidence that comes when you're no longer engaged in the day-to-day struggle of trying to change the unchangeable. You realise that you don't need the parts of your life that you used to justify your anger and frustration that life was so unfair.

The energy that you were spending on struggling against immovable elements in your life can now be applied to altering the things that are changeable. **You have the resources to make changes** available to you, or if you can't, to change the way you think about them.

> I am me. I am myself.
>
> I am a singular, unique human being.
>
> I do not compare myself with anyone else.
>
> I'm not in the wrong place, or with the wrong person.
>
> The way things are is simply just that – the way things are.
>
> I accept them, and in doing so, know that I can change them.
>
> If I want to.

EGO /

The other interesting theme in my husband's New Zealand hunting story is ego. It was his ego that had him pressing on in the wrong direction, even to the extent of questioning his compass! He was more worried about what others would think of him, berating himself that this should not happen to someone with his experience. His ego – the spoilt brat, screaming and stamping his feet – had overtaken his mature sensibilities. And his ego was not happy!

Ego can be the reason why someone won't exercise. They might have a fear about not looking good or not being the best. Ego can be why someone won't start eating better, because they may feel that by doing so they're admitting they've been wrong and that those who are asking them to change were right.

For many people, while they *know* what needs to be done, its more than their pride can swallow to take that first step towards change.

Your ego can often hold you back from acceptance and the personal growth that comes from moving forward. By way of example, I recently became interested in CrossFit, the tough, military-style training that has a reputation for short but incredibly demanding workouts. Now, I like to try new training regimes, but because of my public persona as *The Biggest Loser* trainer people expect me to be super fit and able to do anything physical. Which, I can assure you, isn't always the case.

If I hadn't kept my ego in check, I would never have experienced CrossFit, because the embarrassment of falling short of the expectations others had of me would have been too much. The same can be said of the sessions with my personal trainer, Joey, which have been equally rewarding. And let me tell you, my ego took a beating in some of those workouts; there was a fair amount of blood, sweat, tears and dignity being left on the gym floor!

My immersion in a whole new world of different training, **being challenged** and having my arse kicked by a trainer, has given me **a new philosophy and attitude to physical exertion**.

Knowing that my weaknesses would be exposed *almost* allowed my ego to stop me from experiencing some of the best training I've ever had! Thankfully, I kept it in check and accepted my situation.

I said to Joey, 'I figure, what is there to really be scared of? I mean, what's the worst that can happen? I run out of gas? If I can't keep going . . . I fall over. That's it. I'm not going to die. If others think less of me, that's not my issue.'

Having this realisation made me fearless with my training. It's actually been really empowering.

Accepting that I won't be the fastest or the strongest or the fittest doesn't actually matter because I'm **moving forward**. I'm having a go. It's so bloody liberating and I end up going into a training session totally unfazed!

This fearlessness is available to *anyone* who is prepared to jettison their ego.

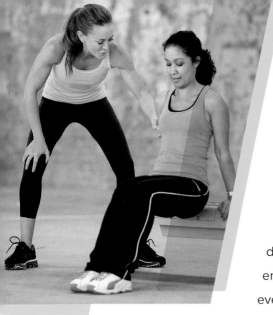

If your actions are motivated by concern about what others think, or worrying about being made to look silly, then your personal development is destined to remain at a standstill. **Trust me!** All of these things are gonna happen regardless! You may as well keep moving and learn along the way.

Not allowing your ego to determine your actions doesn't have to be about health and fitness. Quietening your ego at work, in relationships and in your everyday life will also open new possibilities.

With CONSCIENCE comes SELF-RESPECT.

With SELF-RESPECT comes ACKNOWLEDGEMENT.

With ACKNOWLEDGEMENT comes ACCEPTANCE.

With ACCEPTANCE comes SELF-LOVE.

CONSCIENCE /

The last notion that comes from my husband's story is the value of listening to your conscience – that quiet voice from within. In my husband's case, his conscience was the voice of reason. The voice that was able to look beyond just himself and see the bigger picture.

It was this voice that allowed him to look from a completely different perspective on the reality of his situation, to **acknowledge the changes that needed to be made**, and even to enjoy a strange sense of gratification that he was now back to moving forward.

We all have this voice within us. It's the one that is often drowned out by ego, but is still always there, quiet and unwavering. Some people call it gut instinct; others call it their inner spirit. Either way, it's there. In all of us.

Our conscience guides us. Listen to it.

This is the voice that protects us from comparisons, guilt, negative judgements, living in the past, living in fear, being angry and doing dumb things. It is the voice that gives us courage, self-belief in ourselves and belief in others, respect, wisdom, and a sense of the greater good.

These are the kinds of things that the voice – your conscience – says:

- 'I never drink and drive.'
- 'I don't eat caged chickens.'
- 'I don't use bad language in front of my kids.'
- 'I don't abuse my body because I want to be around to see my grandchildren grow up.'
- 'I don't cheat in business.'

These are just examples, and you will have your own, but note that they aren't 'I will train three times a week' or 'I will go to cooking classes next month'. They are more fundamental than that. They are principles – notions by which you live your life. They are powerful things and it is your conscience that regulates them.

OUR BODIES ARE PERFECT /

It is from a place of 'conscience', not ego, that we can fully embrace the notion of our perfect bodies. Because at the end of the day, our bodies are perfect just the way they are. With all their flaws and imperfections, they are **the perfect manifestation of what we have done to them** – how we have nourished them, exercised them, used them – since we were born.

Our physical selves are merely a reflection of how we have treated our skin, bones, muscles and connective tissue over the years. We have responded perfectly to the influences of our nutrition, lifestyle and environment, but here's the thing – **you can change your body by giving it different messages.**

So while we might think that we're stuck with a certain physical body, we're not. Now I'm not talking about morphing from a classic pear shape to a

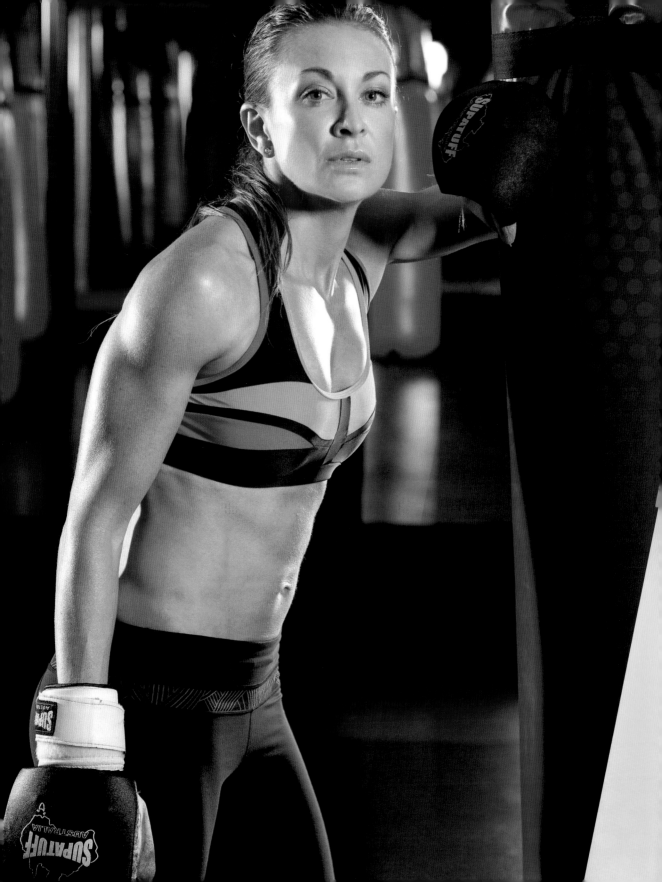

Your body does not make its own decisions.
What you decide, your body will respond to.

cat-walk model here. What I am saying is that a large part of our health and how we look is not so much the genes we were born with, but what we've done with them since.

Nothing happens overnight here. Your body is a long time in the making, and it's not quick to change. But change it will, because your body is perfect. It responds perfectly to what you tell it to do.

Eat more calories than you burn off, and your body will store them and you'll get bigger. Cut down on the calories and up your energy expenditure, and it will get smaller again. It will simply do as it's told, and **you are the one who's giving out the instructions**.

Start training with weights, and not only will your muscles strengthen to compensate, but your bones will become bigger and more dense. Follow the workouts in this book and your core strength will improve, as will your heart and lung functions.

Try playing this game with yourself when your body's complaining mid-workout and you're wishing you kissed your husband goodbye because quite clearly you'll never see him again! Tell yourself of your body's perfection when, on the face of it, it seems to be displaying imperfection.

When you're sprinting intervals on the treadmill and sucking in the big ones, remind yourself that far from your body *failing* to cope, **it's responding exactly as it should to the influences you're exerting on it**.

By increasing your rate of breathing, your body is amping up the oxygen flow to fuel your muscles as well as combining that oxygen with other fuels like glycogen and stored body fat. It needs to get this fuel to hungry muscles faster, so it has responded by cranking up your heart rate express-delivering fuel all around your body – every artery, vein and capillary. Looked at like that, your body is nothing short of amazing.

This adaptation principle is a basic tenet of the survival of our species. The perfect machines that are our bodies were always designed to change and adapt to their circumstances and surroundings.

EPIGENETICS – BEYOND YOUR DNA

The unravelling of the human genome has presented us with some fascinating insights about our bodies, in particular the science of epigenetics.

I first came across epigenetics when I met Professor Paul Taylor on the set of *The Biggest Loser.* He told me about the relationship between chronological age and biological age, and about the way our genes are expressed through our lifestyle choices. I was gobsmacked to learn that how we live our lives can change how our genes express themselves, which can, in turn, affect the genes of our children and grandchildren.

The unborn female foetus develops her own eggs between 16 and 20 weeks. These are the only eggs she will *ever make.* The lifestyle choices that are made by her pregnant mother at this critical time will, through the way her genes express themselves, affect her daughter, but also her grandchildren and even later generations.

Let me put this in context. The child produced by a couple when they are both overweight and in poor health at conception would be different to the child that they would have produced if they were both fit and healthy at conception – *even though the parents' genes were the same.* Now THAT is a powerful message!

Professor Taylor explained that since we have unravelled the human genome, scientists have discovered that the genetic hardwiring of our physical selves is not all-encompassing. In fact, only around 40 per cent of our physical-ity is genetically predetermined; the remaining 60 per cent is affected by our lifestyles – what we eat, and whether or not we exercise.

The science of epigenetics is about this 60 per cent of ourselves that we can change, which is the *genetic expression* of our genes rather than our genetic make-up itself. It's about how our treatment of our genes has influenced the way they express themselves and produced the current human form that we have today.

What epigenetic research is telling us is that our genes themselves are not wholly responsible for our physical characteristics. It studies the changes in our physical properties that are caused by mechanisms *over and above* our underlying DNA sequence. **So it's not the cards you are dealt, but how you play them.**

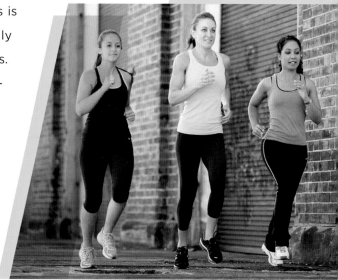

Epigenomes act a bit like a dimmer switch; they sit on top of our genes, and effectively tell them which genetic characteristics to switch on, and which to switch off, which to increase and which to diminish. So they not only determine whether or not certain genes express themselves, they also tell them *to what extent* that expression should happen.

And that 'dimming up, dimming down' ability is all **controlled by us, by how we live our lives**. It means we can change our propensity to disease and to obesity, even the way we look, by changing our diet, our exercise habits and our environment.

One thing that doesn't change, though, is our DNA sequence itself. We can't change this sequence because it's hardwired into our system. We can only change our epigenetics: how our genes express themselves.

Obviously, if we could switch off the genes that give us a propensity to develop cancer or obesity, or at least 'dim' them, there would be enormous benefits for us, which is why scientists are now getting really interested in epigenetic research.

If there is one thing that every contestant on *The Biggest Loser* has told me, without exception, it is that they have 'tried everything, but nothing's worked' in their quest for a healthy weight. And yet we managed to get weight off all of them – without exception. Does that mean they left their fat genes at the front door? No. Did we change their DNA sequence? No. They just altered the genetic expression of their genes.

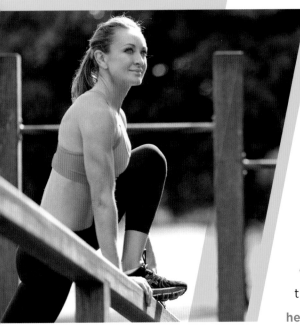

Even though it takes time to see the result of changes in your diet, exercise and environment, the change to your epigenome – and therefore your genetic expression – is *immediate.* Never think that the changes you've made to your lifestyle haven't made a difference – they have.

So **every single choice you make** – to have a glass of water instead of a can of soft drink, or power-walk the dog instead of standing chatting to other dog owners – **improves your overall health and wellbeing** straightaway!

EXERCISE AND LONGEVITY

The cellular changes that we make through altering our diet and exercise patterns aren't short-term propositions, provided we are consistent. Being an exerciser has got more benefits than improved physiology and better brain function. **Best bodies are generally around a lot longer than those that aren't so well looked after.** Let's be honest: you don't see many morbidly obese people who are in their 80s and 90s. They just don't exist.

There have been several studies that demonstrate this fact, but one in particular makes the point loud and clear. It found that a 65-year-old regular exerciser can expect an additional 12.7 years of healthy life on the planet. And if he or she happens to be a highly active 65-year-old, then you can add another 5.7 years on top of that. Incredible! That's over 18 years!

And having been an advocate of vigorous exercise all my life (it's got me caught up in a lot of debate on more than one occasion by naysayers, but, hey, I can handle it), I was stoked to see that going a bit harder in your workouts makes a difference – more than five years difference in fact!

But here's the clincher for me – the additional years of life are *disability free.* The same study found that even if you've done bugger all for most of your life, then you start exercising at a ripe 50 years of age, getting yourself on a relatively intense program like the ones in this book, then you can still expect an additional 3.7 years of disability-free life.

So, if you ever need a bit of extra motivation, **think about all the extra time you'll be able to spend with your kids and grandkids**.

A STORY ABOUT PERCEPTION /

This is a modern parable that originated in naval circles that shows how reality and perception can sometimes work against each other.

Two battleships assigned to a training squadron had been at sea on manoeuvres in heavy weather for several days. As night fell the visibility was poor, with patchy fog, so the captain of one of the ships remained on the bridge keeping an eye on all activities.

Shortly after dark, the lookout on the wing of the bridge reported, 'Light, bearing on the starboard bow.'

'Is it steady or moving astern?' the captain called out.

'Steady, captain,' came the reply, meaning they were on a direct collision course with the ship.

The captain then called to the signalman, 'Signal that ship: we are on a collision course; advise you to change course 20 degrees.'

Back came a signal, 'Advisable for you to change course 20 degrees.'

The captain said, 'Send: I'm captain; change course 20 degrees.'

'I'm a seaman second class,' came the reply. 'You had better change course 20 degrees.'

By that time the captain was furious. He spat out, 'Send: I'm a battleship. Change course 20 degrees.'

Back came the flashing light, 'I'm a lighthouse.'

The ship changed course.

I love how this story gives the reader, as well as the captain, a quick, sharp donk on the head about how **the reality of a situation can clash with our perception** of it.

Just like the captain of the battleship, we too can allow our perception of reality to limit our thinking, We can find ourselves lost in a fog of believing that we are stuck with things the way they are, based on our narrow perceptions, and that there's no opportunity to change them! And the longer we leave ourselves in this fog of perception, the more these feelings and emotions make it thicker and murkier, and those thoughts of 'this is the way it is' become more and more concrete.

Over the past 20 years, I have worked with thousands of women and men who have broken themselves against their lighthouses so many times that they feel they are literally in a thousand pieces. The making and breaking of promises has left them feeling shattered and disillusioned.

I know, as intrinsically we all probably do, that life doesn't have to be that way. At the end of the day, **we all have the opportunity to make changes** in our lives. And it's not just about food and exercise. I made the point in my first book, *Crunch Time,* that exploring new directions for yourself, getting healthy, fitter or losing weight starts with the way in which you choose to think. **You must change your perception to change your body**.

It's almost a cliché, but a healthy mind really is crucial to a healthy body. Having clarity in your thinking and embracing possibilities will lead to positive outcomes.

PRINCIPLES /

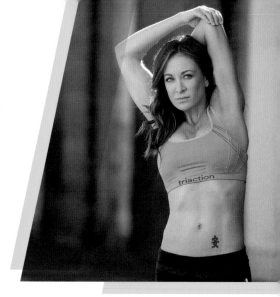

When I start training a client I like to ask them early in the relationship if they are a man or woman of their word. Most of them quickly leap to their own defence – 'Yes, I am! Of course I am!' – and offer up an opinion of themselves that establishes them as a person of honour and principles.

Yet when it comes to crunch time, often they are not. They can't stick to the eating plan I gave them, even though they said they would. They don't do their training homework, even though they promised to. It is a totally different ball game when it comes time to walk the walk, not just talk the talk (as it is for many of us).

What they don't realise is that they have more to gain by being straight with me in the first place, realising that when it comes to diet and exercise they tend not to be men or women of their word, and then going through some introspection to uncover the reasons *why* they aren't, and determine what they would like to do about it.

When this happens they have the opportunity to be *guided* by their light-houses – their principles – instead of sailing into them, to re-establish and create principles.

You **begin to move forward** because you've set your lighthouses up to light your way. There are things that you are prepared to do, and there are things that you aren't prepared to do because they breach the principles that guide your life.

You now start to understand things that you never knew before, and you **start seeing things differently**. Things about your environment, your career, your family, yourself. Interestingly, you can also look back over past events with fresh eyes, and see different outcomes, perhaps even know now that you would have acted very differently.

CINDY'S STORY

While pregnant with my son, I bought a gorgeous dress to wear to an upcoming wedding. My son was born in January 2011 and the wedding was December 2011 – surely I would be able to fit into my new size 8 dress by then? Um, no. A few weeks before the wedding I tried on my new dress. Verdict – a big fat fail. Literally.

During my pregnancy I managed to put on 20 kilograms (no thanks to the crazy concoction of medication I was on at the time for my lupus). I assumed that I would just naturally lose the weight after the baby was born, but that was definitely not the case.

In the end I had to wear a different dress to the wedding, one that I wore three months after my son was born and while I was still breastfeeding – let's just say that the dress was quite a 'comfortable' fit.

By the time of my son's first birthday I was still carrying extra weight and couldn't fit into my jeans for his party. That was it for me. Something had to change.

I was a fan of *The Biggest Loser* and so turned to Michelle's program. The rest is history! I managed to lose the excess baby weight and reached my goal of 50 kilograms. I could fit into my clothes again!

The best thing has been that I have maintained my weight loss and my new lifestyle has had a big impact on my health. My high blood pressure, caused by the lupus, has come right down, as have my blood sugar and cholesterol levels.

Initially it was tricky to manage family, work, health, life and the program. But after a few weeks I found a balance. It helped that Michelle's recipes are so quick and easy. I definitely found a new appreciation for food and cooking.

Michelle's method is so much more than a nutrition and fitness program – it also focuses on the mind and the reasons why we think and act in certain ways. Michelle's program helped me become much more consistent in my actions and choices.

I've had lots of positive feedback from family and friends regarding the way I now look. More importantly, I have loved seeing and feeling myself improve.

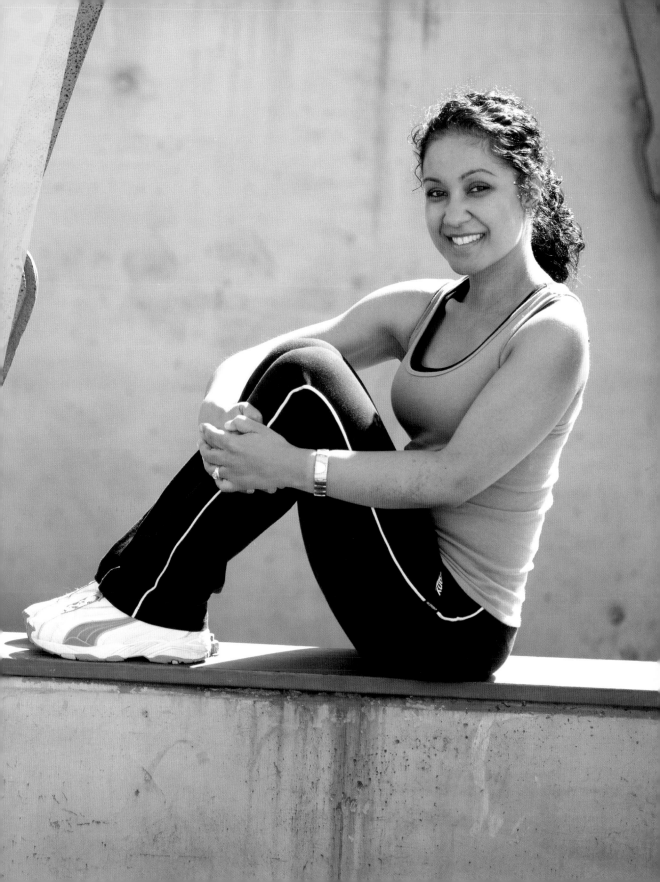

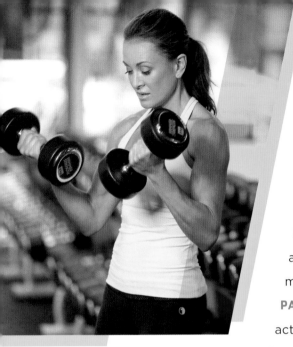

THE PRINCIPLES LIST /

Draw up a list with three parts.

PART 1 / Make the first part your personal principles. What are the **principles** that you wish to live your life by? These could be honesty, loyalty, and respect, but these are quite generic concepts. Drill down and qualify them, e.g. I will be honest about my food intake to my family, my trainer and myself.

PART 2 / The second part should be **actions**. What actions will you need to take to guarantee that you live up to the principles in the first column? Be very descriptive in your action list, making sure to get down to specifics.

PART 3 / The last part should list **past events** that would have had different outcomes had you used those actions to stick to your principles.

PRINCIPLES LIST EXAMPLE 1

PRINCIPLE / To be honest and accountable with myself about my nutrition and my exercise.

ACTION / I eat more than I admit to myself. I need to be honest about the excuses I make around exercise and eating healthily. I will write down all of my excuses, cross off the ones that are ridiculous and find solutions to those that are genuine.

PAST EVENT / Last weekend I ordered a large pizza and garlic bread for myself before I went out to dinner with friends. I ordered fish and salad in front of them in an attempt to look like I was being healthy.

This wasn't a reflection of my new stated principles and I let myself down because I wasn't being honest with my friends, or myself. This led me to feel that I was a failure and consequently I hated myself. I can NOW see that if I had stuck to my principle not only would I NOT be feel these things, I would actually feel the exact opposite! I would have questioned my choices and not eaten in private to avoid accountability.

PRINCIPLES LIST EXAMPLE 2

PRINCIPLE / To respect my loved ones and understand that they love me.

ACTION / I feel that I need to have more respect for my relationship with my husband, as I tend to take my anxiety about my weight problems out on him. The disrespect that I feel for myself is a mirror image of how I treat him. Next time he suggests that we go for a walk, or have a cup of tea instead of eating a block of chocolate, I want to respect that he is expressing love for me, not denying me what I want. I also don't want to act out in rebellion. I can see that I am doing that just to hurt him, but I know that I am hurting me too.

PAST EVENT / On Tuesday night I asked my husband to go to the shop to buy me a packet of biscuits. He refused saying that they aren't really what I want to be eating as I'd only just said that day that I wanted to lose some weight. I then lost my temper, stormed up to the shop and bought not one but three packets of biscuits out of spite. I proceeded to eat the lot in a foul mood. I can see now that if I had applied my new principle, then I would not be resenting him and feeling upset, and I would not have upset him too. We might have even gone for a walk instead, which would have strengthened our relationship. And that's without the regret of the gazillion calories I just inhaled!

This kind of work takes guts. To write down a set of principles is not easy, but it's still a lot easier than living by them! Especially because when you are writing them you might be thinking 'Jeez, I really don't know if I can live up to these for the rest of my life!' Be prepared to fail, but don't let it stop you from doing the drill. Trust me. If you didn't fail, we'd all be calling you the next Messiah and bowing down at your sandal-wearing feet.

That said, don't be a hypocrite and have all these principles stuck on sticky notes all over your fridge and bathroom mirror, and not live by any of them! It's about being conscious of what's going on around and within you, seeing the potential to screw up, and **making measured thoughtful choices**. Sometimes you screw up. It's called being human. The big question is what you do afterwards. Do you learn the lesson? Instead of completely breaking yourself over that lighthouse, do you feel the warning hit and steer in another direction?

Many people will glaze over when I talk about these kinds of drills thinking 'Yeah, yeah, I know where she's going here. I get it. Now lets get onto the diet and exercise bit'.

To me this is like someone who plays tennis just once a week signing themselves up for the state championships in order to make a better impression on their mates. No matter how much positive thinking this person does, they will get slaughtered!

It's the same with health and fitness. You cannot violate, ignore or take shortcuts in the natural order of things. Attempting to hunt down the shortcut will result in disappointment and disenchantment.

Yo-yo dieters are the classic short-cutters. Generally speaking, they are all about the quick fix rather than the slow burn.

Significant changes to lifestyle take time and planning, but it is the only way that offers lasting results.

WHAT DO YOU WANT?

This shouldn't be a hard question, but lots of people baulk when I ask it. Most of us are clear on what we *don't* want, but often struggle when we try and understand exactly what it is we *do* want.

I often hear things put in negative terms, such as, 'I don't want to be this weight anymore' or 'I'm sick and tired of feeling sick and tired'. But believe me, it makes a great difference if you can formulate changes you want to make in a positive way.

So first grab a pen and a piece of paper and write a list, and be as specific as you can.

This is a really good drill because it helps us set goals that are important to us – positive changes we want to achieve and targets that can help us keep motivated and striving to be the best we can.

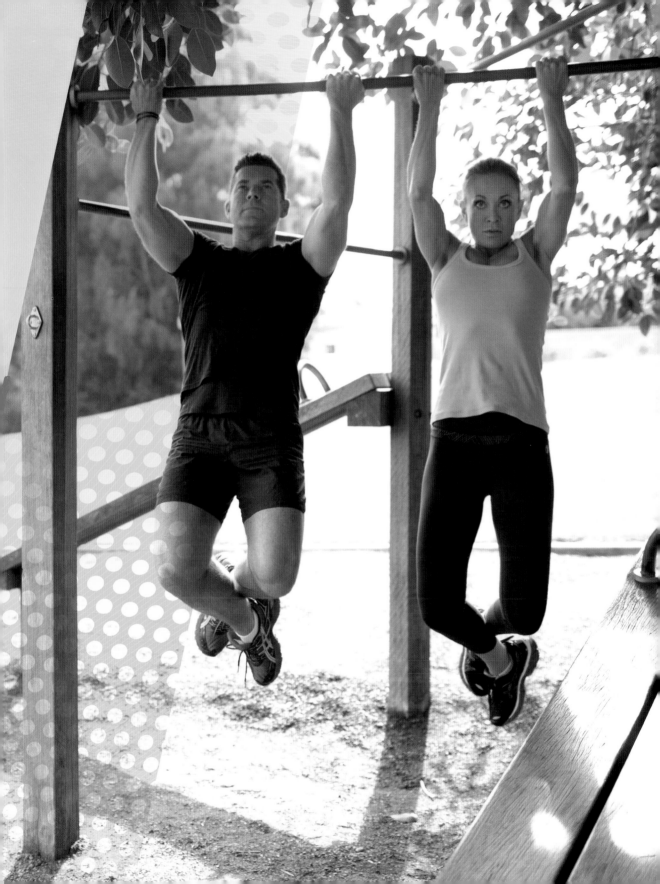

LIST OF WANTS EXAMPLE

- I want to be able to run 5 kilometres nonstop.
- I want to lose my love handles and feel slimmer before the first day of spring.
- I want to team up with my daughter so we can both lose 5 kilos each before her wedding.
- I want to see what improvements I can make to my triathlon times in two months.
- I want to be able to do ten full push-ups on my toes without stopping.
- I want to fit back into my wedding dress before Christmas.
- I want to play touch footy again next season and feel confident running out on the field.
- I want to learn how to eat healthily and improve my cooking skills.

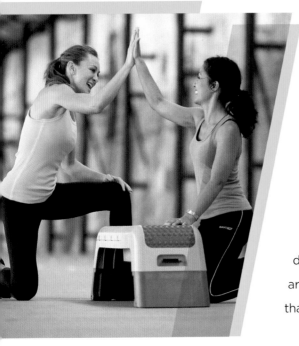

Now you need to ask yourself: What excuses have I used to stop me from achieving these goals in the past?

Be ruthless! Write down as many excuses as you can think of that you have used or are likely to use. (I have a female client who I have worked with for over six months and she can still come up with over 20 excuses!)

When you have all these excuses written down, delete the ridiculous ones (come on – some of them are ridiculous!), and then find solutions to the ones that are left by formulating specific action plans.

These drills may seem a bit tedious, and you might be inclined to gloss over them. **But be warned!** If you're the type of person that tends to be hot and cold, or maybe a yo-yo dieter, then this is where you are *always* going wrong.

ALL-OR-NOTHING THINKING /

People who want to rush in and get started on lifestyle changes without the proper preparation are, in my experience, the ones that are most likely to fail. The 'I want it all and I want it now' mentality of always looking for the shortcut to reach a goal as fast as possible simply doesn't have the success rate of the more **measured, calculated approach needed for profound changes**.

For this reason, my online personal-training and weight loss program, the '12 Week Body Transformation', insists that participants go through my 'pre-season tasks'. I insist they do this because I know it *works,* something that is backed up by research conducted by Professor Susan Byrne, a psychologist from the University of Western Australia.

She did an interesting study that highlighted the potential pitfalls of what she calls 'dichotomous thinking' – the all-or-nothing, black-and-white approach to life.

People who charged into their weight-loss journeys in this all-or-nothing frame of mind generally set unrealistic goals and imposed strict diet and exercise plans on themselves. But these plans are hard to keep to (unless you're stuck in *The Biggest Loser* house with me kicking your butt every day), and Professor Byrne found that such people were more likely to chuck the whole thing in and go back to unhealthy eating at the slightest provocation – even if they had just a single lapse.

The slow-burners who didn't have this dichotomous thinking style turned out, in contrast, to be happier with a modest weight loss, even if it fell short of their goal. But they were also more likely to carry on eating well and exercising regularly, having accepted that, while they may not yet have reached their target, they were still better off than when they started.

So be aware that **your long-term outcome is likely to be affected by your mindset at the get-go**. If you put in the effort at the preparation stage you are much more likely to reach all your goals. So take your time – and do the drills!

Setting the groundwork, getting your head in the right place and putting a plan together is the best way to start making lasting changes.

SLEEP /

Sleep is a crucial component in getting us in a positive mental space to make changes. A good night's sleep is essential, not just to feeling sufficiently energised for a training session, but to avoid that dragging-your-arse-around feeling that follows an unsettled night between the sheets.

If you find yourself struggling to get a good night's sleep, then you are ingood company. Around 1.5 million Australians suffer from sleep disorders that's about 9 per cent of the population!

We know that **exercise, particularly aerobic exercise, contributes to a good night's sleep**. When I was working as a group fitness instructor I would often teach four, five, sometimes six high-energy one-hour classes in a day, and in those days, let me tell you, I was at one with my mattress for nine hours straight. (Apparently scientists are still unclear as to why this is, but all they have to do is ask!)

There is also a correlation between fatigue and our blood sugar levels. Elevated blood sugar levels can increase our potential to accumulate fat. And if you're in the market to drop a couple of kilos, you'll be interested to know that your levels of the appetite-suppressing hormone leptin are reduced when you are tired. And to make matters worse, your levels of appetite-stimulating hormone ghrelin are *increased*, which may lead to overeating.

There is a link between being tired and being stressed, and when we're stressed things go wrong. Our adrenal glands pump out a whole bunch of hormones, one of which is cortisol. Cortisol temporarily puts your non-essential bodily functions on hold and prompts a glucose-fest, spraying it all through your body. The brain picks up most of it to deal with the crisis at hand, but the rest ends up in the bloodstream. Which results in fat. Around your middle.

The other great deceiver in the elusive world of 'A Good Night's Sleep' is alcohol. We often think that a night on the turps will guarantee a good night's sleep because we pass out the moment we lie down.

But that isn't actually a good thing. If you fall asleep too quickly it's a sign of sleep deprivation. Ideally you **should take around ten to fifteen minutes to doze off**, but never less than five minutes.

Alcohol will often see you comatose in five *seconds*, and although you go into a deep sleep straightaway this usually only lasts for a couple of hours. After that your sleep pattern becomes distorted, with the deep sessions that we would normally experience every 90 minutes or so being replaced with long periods of light, restless sleep.

MY SLEEP TIPS

1. Never fall asleep on the couch. If you start to feel tired, go to bed.
2. There are only two things that should happen in the bedroom, and one of them is sleeping. And neither of them includes phones, iPads, laptops or televisions and the like. These things should stay in the lounge.
3. Get the room temperature right. Our brains try to achieve a particular (cooler) body temperature when we sleep, and if our environment is much warmer or colder we will generally wake up. It's hard to recommend the optimum temperature, but for most people it wil be around 18–22 degrees centigrade.
4. Think of your bedroom as a cave – very quiet, quite cool and black when the lights are off. Even the smallest ray of light can turn off a neural switch in your brain, causing a drop in the chemicals that induce sleep, so keep the digital alarm clock out of sight. Besides, checking the time and worrying about how many hours sleep you have left is destructive.
5. Even though your bedroom should be cool, your hands and feet shouldn't be cold.
6. No caffeine after 3.00 p.m.

7. Napping is okay, but never closer than eight hours before you got to bed, and not for more than 20–30 minutes.

8. Try and go to bed and get up at the same time every day, including at the weekend.

9. Do your vigorous exercise in the morning. A gut-buster before you go to bed will mean you're fired up and will delay your drifting off. By contrast, yoga, tai chi and relaxation classes are good pre-bed training routines.

10. Eat early, and light. We've all been there, tossing and turning feeling like we've swallowed a pillow. Big, late meals will always make for an unsettled night, and also contribute to weight gain.

11. Keep the lights low before you go to bed as this stimulates the production of melatonin, the sleep-inducing hormone. Swap a couple of bulbs for 15 watts and use those lights around the house before bedtime.

12. As with pretty much everything when it comes to smoking, it is . . . actually, I can't even be bothered talking about it. Dumb, dumb, dumb.

13. A recent survey showed that 42 per cent of pet owners let their pets sleep with them, which is especially weird when the same survey showed that only 23 per cent of respondents let their children sleep with them. Need I say more?

14. If you suffer with back problems and they wake you up, try sleeping with a pillow between your legs if you sleep on your side, or behind your knees if you sleep on your back.

15. Sleeping pills are a last resort, and I recommend you try everything on this list before you go down that path. If your sleeplessness is persistent, it's time to dig deeper for the cause. Have a good chat to your doctor, or see a sleep therapist.

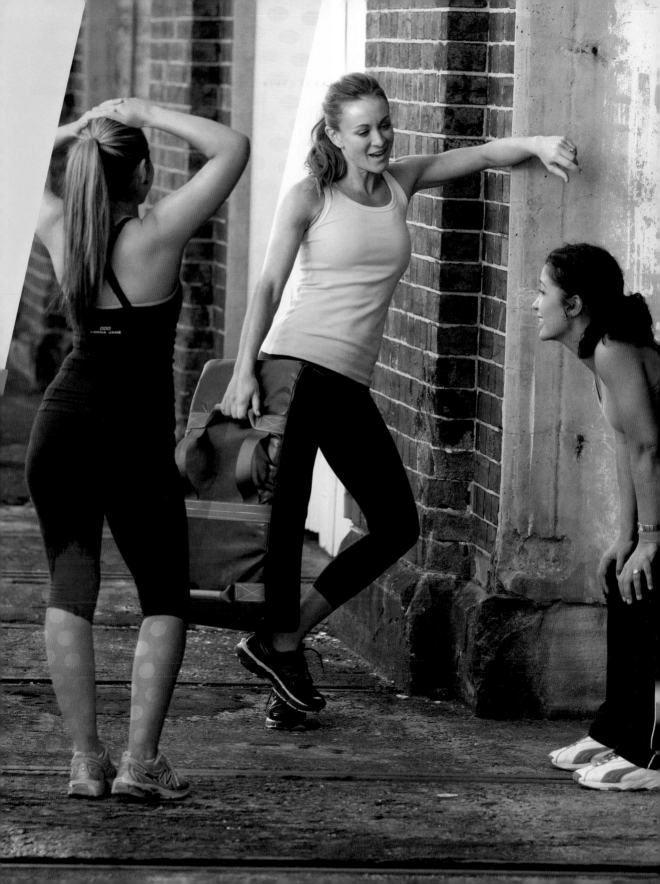

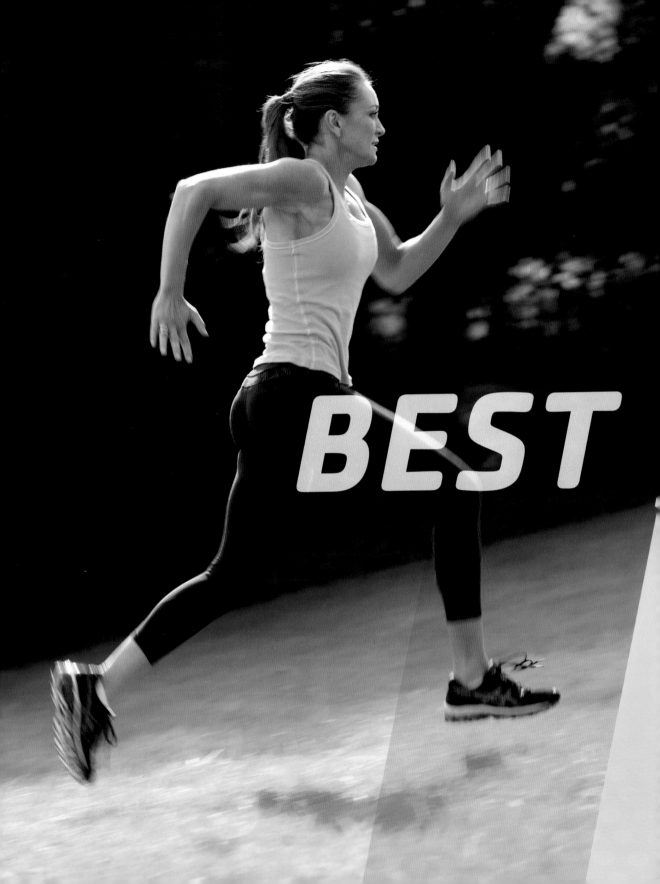

training

Our bodies are designed to move and working out is essential to achieving your best body. These exercises are amazing because they are 'super compound' – the ultimate time effective, total body exercise therapy! These are the exercises I do myself, arranged in the workouts that I use to get in the best possible shape.

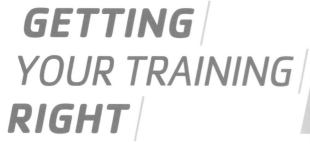

GETTING YOUR TRAINING RIGHT

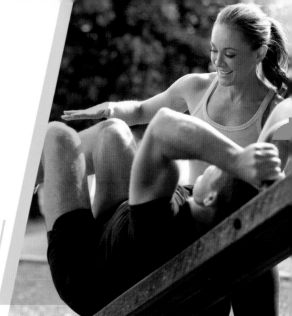

Your best body is able to do just about anything really well:

- From running a race to moving heavy furniture
- From riding a bike to playing with your kids in the backyard
- From enjoying a game of golf to changing a car tyre
- From digging the garden to walking the dog

Such activities are part of our lives today, so we need to stay active, keep mobile and move well for a long period of time (I'm talking into your 80s) to really get the most out of life.

This book, like my others, contains training methods that offer **overall fitness, strength and agility**. I've always mixed up my training, and I've always been a big believer in circuits and intervals because I know they work and give fast results. They expose you to multiple exercise modalities, which in turn will give you the best possible outcome – your best body.

And with everybody's number-one excuse being 'time poor', and wanting fast measurable results, the type of training I set out in this book comes into its own. Plus it stops the bitching about getting bored easily because of the constant variety and combinations of exercises!

My personal philosophy has always been that your strength will be in knowing your weaknesses. With this kind of training, your weaknesses will be exposed in the physical sense. By always doing what you are good at or what you like all the time, you can cause imbalances, injuries, get stale or, worse yet, never discover your full potential!

Ignoring your weaknesses, and always playing to your strengths, will leave you exposed to mediocrity and you'll never achieve the best possible version of yourself, physically, mentally, and, yes – slipping on my kaftan and burning some incense – dare I say it, even spiritually.

But it's not always easy to address your weaknesses when your ego has a habit of getting in the way of you moving forward. This is a huge reason why many people choose not to exercise at all, preferring to do what I call 'staying safe on the sidelines', for fear of failure.

Mentally, however, it is a great loss. You never get a chance to be challenged, to feel a little lost, scared or nervous. Having to dig deep, when you are on your knees thinking 'I don't know if I can get up', undoubtedly **builds strength of character, integrity and a quietly humbling sense of resolve**. This, in turn, allows you to appreciate others and their achievements, and can foster a real sense of camaraderie when training in a group. These characteristics and experiences are better than a fit strong body any day, but if you're lucky enough to have both? Empowering!

VISIT YOUR DOCTOR /

If you haven't been to see your doctor recently, now would be a good time to go. Apart from the benefit of keeping a close eye on your health – which, since you have bought this book, is evidently something you are interested in – it's also good to benchmark where you're at physiologically with some tests.

Many of the changes that will happen to you by following the diet and exercise plans in this book are subtle, and require pathology if you are to see them. Triglycerides, for example, the storage form of fat, can only be measured through a blood test, but it's important that they are kept at the correct levels.

Some of the benchmarks you can measure yourself, and while they are less technical, they are nonetheless important. For me, there are two measurements that should always be at the very top of your list for checking your progress.

No, not dress size, not even weight. The measurements that I recommend you keep a close eye on are **waist measurement and blood pressure**. These two factors are the most accessible indicators of your health.

Waist measurement sounds a bit simplistic, but it's particularly relevant because it acknowledges the *location* of excess fat on our bodies, which a key indicator of our likelihood of developing chronic diseases that, let me tell you, you just don't want to acquire.

WAIST MEASUREMENT (cm) AND RISK OF HEART DISEASE

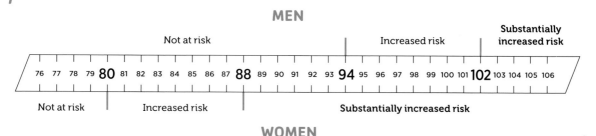

Source: Queensland Department of Local Government, Sport and Recreation 2008

Unlike Body Mass Index (BMI) (which gets an unfair slagging from many people because it doesn't necessarily apply to everyone, even though for my money it is a good wake-up call), waist measurement is particularly good because it works irrespective of your height, weight, age, gender, race, build, whatever. And it's as simple as wrapping a tape around your middle.

Blood pressure, while a little more technical, is also easy to monitor. You might be surprised to learn that your local chemist probably sells blood pressure machines for not a lot of money, so it too is a very accessible measurement. It can be an early indication of potential health issues, and so monitoring our blood pressure gives us the opportunity to do something about it before chronic illness develops.

BLOOD PRESSURE TABLE

Guide to adult blood pressure ranges

Top number (systolic) mm of mercury	Bottom number (diastolic) mm of mercury	Diagnosis	Action
below 120	below 80	Normal	Ideal adult range – keep making healthy diet and exercise choices!
120–139	80–89	Pre-hypertension	Make conscious changes to your diet and activity levels, and monitor closely
140–159	90–99	Stage 1 hypertension	Make conscious changes to your diet and activity levels, and if your blood pressure has not reduced in six months consult your doctor
160 +	100 +	Stage 2 hypertension	Ring and make an appointment with your doctor today

CARDIO TRAINING

I've been a cardio trainer all my life, and I don't think there's ever been a time in my life that I didn't rely on it as a fantastic heart-strengthening, mood-elevating, fat-burning *weapon*!

For most of us, our introduction to exercise was based around cardio activity. School sports, athletics, and generally running around the place all formed the basis of our early exposure to exercise. Unfortunately we can sometimes overlook it as we get older.

But **cardio training has so many benefits** that it would be fair to say you won't get the full benefit of your training regime unless cardio is a part of it. Far from overlooking it, I have included plenty of cardio exercises in the programs in this book that will get your heart pumping like crazy.

Your heart is not the only beneficiary of cardio training. Our lungs improve their capacity to bring oxygen into our bodies, and our vascular system improves to allow that oxygen to be transported to our muscles more efficiently. We sometimes forget that our muscles, like our heart, are organs too, organs that have a vital role in our day-to-day physiological functions. They are designed to move. **We are designed to move** – that is the function of our muscles, and therefore the natural action of a healthy body.

Muscles convert chemical energy into mechanical energy. It's this mechanical energy that not only contracts muscles to allow your body to move, but also provides the force that pushes substances through your body. So, even when we don't appear to be in motion, our muscles are busy moving food and blood around – they never stop working.

If your muscles are starting to tire when you're five clicks into a morning run, relax – that's what they're meant to do. If you're sucking in the big ones grinding up a steep hill and your heart's pounding like a Subaru's subwoofer, don't panic – that's what it's meant to do. **Our bodies are perfect**.

Conditioning your body with cardio exercise will also dramatically reduce your risk of heart disease. Don't be fooled into thinking that heart disease is isolated to wheezy old blokes with weight issues – it's the number-one killer of Australians of both sexes.

Cardio training reduces the risk by progressively getting your resting heart rate lower as you get fitter, thereby reducing the heart's daily workload. It also lowers your cholesterol levels and blood pressure, which are both contributors to heart disease when they are elevated.

But importantly, the way that you improve your fitness is critical, particularly if you are starting off from a low fitness base. Jumping onto a treadmill and going as fast as you can for as long as you can really isn't the best way to build fitness.

Trying to improve both the length of your workout and it's intensity all at the same time will quickly see you become disillusioned. Imagine rocking up to the gym knowing that you have to go to your max every workout, or thinking that every workout must be a full hour or longer – yecht! Constantly pushing yourself to your limit doesn't get you rushing back to the treadmill, or doing cartwheels around the bedroom when the alarm goes off on a Sunday morning. This all-or-nothing mentality has been shown to sabotage long-term goals.

Enjoy your training and understand that **gradual, progressive improvement** is best achieved by training for a little longer in some sessions, and a little more intensely in others. Only occasionally should you go for a Personal Best (PB) to measure your progress by upping the ante in both areas.

Even professional athletes separate their training in this way, carefully planning attempts to beat their PBs well in advance with proper preparation.

The fact that improving **your cardiovascular fitness also improves your ability to burn fat** while you're training isn't lost on me. And when do you start to burn fat in your workout? Well, after 20 minutes or so your body will start to use stored body fat as fuel, and the rate at which it will do this is determined by how many beats a minute your heart is working at.

Up until that 20-minute threshold your body will mostly use glycogen, which is a carbohydrate usually stored in your muscles and your liver. But as the glycogen stores run low, your body turns to body fat for fuel.

If fat loss is one of your cardio-training goals, then it makes sense to train when your glycogen stores are at their lowest, which is after a prolonged period of not eating. This is why I **train first thing in the morning**, when I haven't eaten for ten or 12 hours.

The higher your heart rate, the faster fat is being burned. And how high does your heart rate need to be? I use this formula: 220 minus your age, multiplied by 0.75.

The 220 refers to your maximum heartbeats per minute, and subtracting your age from it allows for the gradual reduction in your heart's

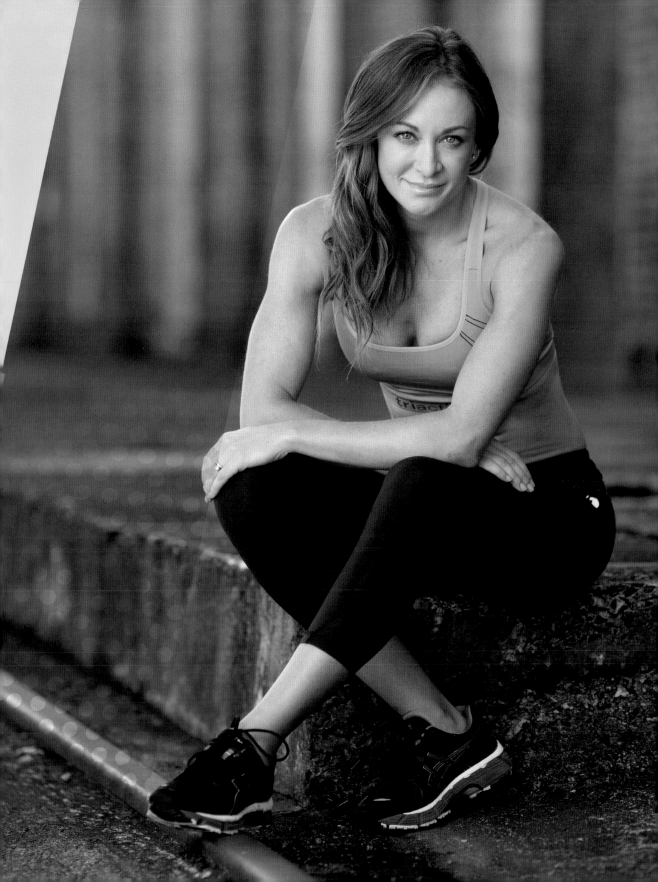

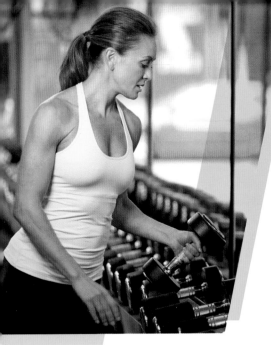

efficiency as you get older. Understand that the 220 is not a scientifically accurate figure, but it is generally recognised as being a close enough estimate for most of us.

Once we start working at around 75 per cent of our maximum heart rate (not an absolute figure, but a rough guide), the energy sources start to change, and we begin to chip away at the fat stored under our skin and around our organs..

Your most valuable tool for this kind of training is a heart rate monitor. Most heart rate monitors allow you to download data from your training sessions so you can keep a record of your journey towards your goal of better health and fitness, but if you prefer to keep written records a diary will be useful.

Getting cardiovascular fitness requires a **gradual increase in your output**. You will need to progressively increase your intensity and/or the length of time that you exercise, so the workout you do on the first day shouldn't look like the workout you're doing six months down the track.

For me, I like to lock in three cardio sessions a week if I need to be keeping my fat levels under control, and one of my favourite fat-loss training methods is interval training. Interval training is where you include regular bursts of high intensity activity during your workout. It's sometimes called 'fartlek' training – which is why I call it interval training!

University tests have shown that interval training stimulates the production of fat-burning hormones called catecholamines, so if fat loss is one of your goals, punch in an interval program next time you're on the cross trainer.

For me, the biggest benefit of cardio training is that is **stimulates the release of the hormone serotonin, the one I call the 'happy hormone'**. No matter how dark a mood I'm in when I start a cardio session, I always walk out with a smile on my face, ready to take on the world.

*Exercise should be an integral part of your life.
Not an after-thought, not the last thing on the list,
but a regular commitment.*

STRENGTH TRAINING /

In the past, exercise types have always fallen into two broad categories – cardio training and strength training. Cardio training by definition targets the cardio-vascular system – heart, lungs, blood supply – by busting your butt on a Sunday morning run, or going crazy in a Body Attack class.

Strength training is mostly associated with weights – sets and reps, pumping iron. It's the grunt and groan of the exercise world, and it's all about getting strong and building muscle.

But for me, strength training has a different role – somewhere in between these two.

Rather than just loading up the dumbbells and straining away, my strength training methods are based around **resistance exercises**, some using weights, others using your bodyweight alone, **put together into groups and performed quickly** with minimal rest.

All of the exercises are compound, meaning that they incorporate more than one muscle group (unlike the isolation exercises frequently used by body-builders). But there the similarity ends because many of my exercises combine muscle groups that have no relation to each other.

There's nothing new about clumping different exercises together to form a 'superset', but traditionally the superset would be based on one muscle (say, your bicep), or opposing muscle groups (first your bicep, then your tricep).

Supersets are still in my repertoire, as are compound weight exercises. But for me the best results come from making exercises 'super compound'. That is, they recruit the majority of the muscles in your body in the same exercise.

So instead of working two opposing muscle groups, my 'super compounds' jump from one body part to the next. From your chest to your legs, then back to your upper body to work your shoulders or back. Or a shoulder exercise that is performed at the same time you are performing a leg exercise. All this happens in the space of one set.

Why is this more effective? Because **the more muscles that are working concurrently, the greater the effort required by your cardiovascular system to keep fuelling them.** The aerobic and anaerobic fuel systems start to overlap, and your body works at its maximum.

I can say that my own training has been taken to a new level since I've been practising 'super compounds' and I can't wait to share this way of training. I got wicked results from it, and you can too.

Strength training delivers so much. A 1994 study by Miriam Nelson published in the *Journal of the American Medical Association* found that 'after a year of strength training twice a week, women's bodies were **15–20 years more youthful**. Without drugs, they regained bone density, became stronger, improved their balance and flexibility, became leaner and trimmer, and were 27 per cent more active. No other program – whether diet, medication or aerobic exercise – has ever achieved comparable results.' The benefits for men too are so well documented it's hardly worth listing them.

But it's a promise that doesn't come cheaply. The strength-training regimes in *Your Best Body* are tough, and there'll be times when you'll be calling me all the names under the sun mid-workout. But don't worry; it's nothing I'm not used to. Just make sure you send me the blessings when you're smokin' a pair of shorts and a singlet the next day.

FUNCTIONAL TRAINING /

Many of the strength exercises in this book are based on functional training principles. Functional training is based around **movements that are replicated in our everyday lives** – picking up things from the floor, bending down to pat your dog.

These exercises started being used in the context of rehabilitation from injuries, but now their broader value is being recognised and they are regularly incorporated into forward-thinking exercise plans.

You may have heard of friends or family who injured themselves performing the most mundane of everyday tasks – perhaps picking up a basket of washing, or crouching down to change the paper in a photocopier. These are the kind of injuries functional training helps protect against.

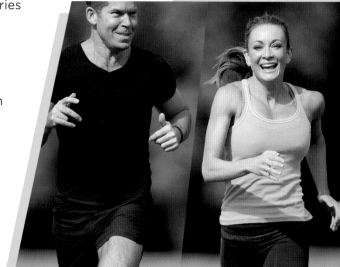

CORE TRAINING /

You'll also notice a lot of core exercises in the programs. Core exercises work the entire **musculature of your midsection**, including the sheets of muscle behind your abdominals, the muscles in your lower back, your glutes and hip flexors, and the muscles around your spine.

The costs of lower-back pain, directly and indirectly, are more than $9 billion a year in Australia, and over $100 billion in the USA. Your best insurance against adding to these numbers is to have a strong, taut core.

Core training isn't all about sit-ups and crunches; it's about exercising the muscles that contribute to your day-to-day health and mobility by stabilising your entire torso from your hips to your shoulders, allowing you to stand up and move in any direction. These muscles extend from your bum to your neck, and they're crucial to health and wellbeing.

BRAIN HEALTH /

After years of training people, hundreds of heart-to-heart conversations with women and men struggling with their weight, and thousands of messages on my websites I'm left in no doubt whatsoever – for most of us to get to the best version of ourselves, it's not about getting our bodies right; it's about getting our heads right.

Getting our heads right requires a healthy brain, with clear thought processes and cognitive functions. Now I'm not taking about finishing Sudoku puzzles faster or going back to uni to do a PhD here (although you could if you wanted to). My interest in brain health – **brain fitness** – is in how it helps to get your head in the right place to make smart lifestyle decisions, stick to them, and feel great in the process.

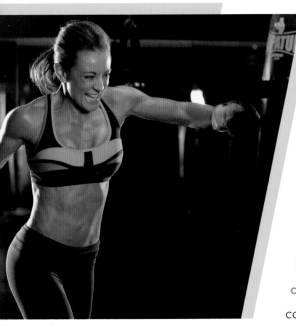

The ability of your brain to re-organise itself by growing new cells, and getting more cells connected to each other is known as brain plasticity. We used to think that adult brains were static, that there was no production of new brain cells after a certain age, but now we know that isn't the case. **Your brain is constantly changing**, growing new cells and creating new connections between existing cells.

TRAINING FOR YOUR BRAIN /

The good news is that we can actually improve our brain plasticity through physical exercise. In fact, **we can do specific exercises to improve specific areas of our brains.**

A 2006 study by the University of Illinois showed that after six months of aerobic exercise a group of 60-plus-year-olds showed a significant increase in volume in some areas of their brains, with the largest increase recorded in the area known as the prefrontal cortex.

This area is particularly important, not only because it is involved in everyday cognitive functions, but also because it has an effect on willpower. Research

> *As the most complex and crucial organ in your body, your brain deserves the best treatment. Make sure it gets the essential nutrients and regular exercise it needs for brain fitness.*

has shown that obese people who struggle with willpower show signs of atrophy in this area of the brain, which diminishes their ability, at a physiological level, to resist tempting foods and cope with the demands of training.

Essentially, our prefrontal cortex is responsible for self-control. It helps us to imagine future outcomes while performing actions in the present. Unfortunately, though, when compared to other areas of the brain, it's actually a bit feeble and tires easily. This is one of the reasons that new year's resolutions fail so spectacularly – the brain requires glucose to function, and the combination of reduced glucose intake through dieting, changed habits and a new exercise routine is usually more than the poor little thing can bear.

The other significant result of the Illinois study was that improvements in brain function were noticed in the participants in just six months. Our brains start to show signs of structural decline in our 30s, so not only did the exercise halt the decline, it actually *reversed it* – and all in just six months.

Exercise can improve the hippocampus area of the brain, which is **critical for memory formation**. This area shrinks in size between one and two per cent a year when we get over 60 – exercise can *grow* it by one to two per cent.

Similarly, we can do specific exercises to activate our cerebellum, located at the back of our heads above the spinal column. The cerebellum is responsible for smooth, coordinated body movements, and we can improve brain plasticity in this area by doing exercises that rely on balance, posture and body weight.

Exercises performed on machines don't activate the cerebellum as much as free-form exercises because the machine prescribes the movement. Free-form exercises require adjustments to your body's position, balance and movement, and so working your brain as well as your muscles. Your body and brain are working together.

We are only just realising the importance of exercise in relation to our cognitive function, particularly as we grow older. Recent studies have shown that we can reduce the risk of developing Alzheimer's disease by an astonishing 50 per cent by incorporating exercise into our lifestyles. That's right, 50 per cent!

HEART HEALTH /

Our hearts deserve special attention because, like our brains, they are critical to our existence. But the relationship between your brain and your heart doesn't end there. Recent studies have also shown **a direct link between brain health and heart health**, with depression being shown to be a key risk factor for cardiovascular disease. And not just a remote link either. Mild depression actually *doubles* the risk of developing heart disease, and severe depression increases the risk *five times*.

Before you start getting all depressed, on the upside remember that anything you do for your brain health – regular aerobic and resistance exercise, plenty of omega-3s and folic acid, minimising saturated fats – equally benefits your heart, so you're covering both bases.

TRAINING FOR A HEALTHY HEART /

The best way to connect with your heart when you're training is to know what it's doing, and the best way to do that is by using a heart rate monitor (HRM). I'm a big fan of HRMs for a few reasons, but mainly because I can accurately monitor the intensity at which I'm training without having to rely on my 'perceived rate of exertion'. I like to try lots of different types of exercise and knowing how my heart is responding to them is, for me, invaluable. I like to be able to track the number of calories I've burned during my workouts, but I also use my HRM as a physiological reference by:

- Training until a certain number of calories are burned
- Using it as an recovery indicator between sets in the weight room
- Targeting a specific heart rate during training.

Most HRMs have a function that allows you to retrieve and store historic data from previous workouts, and even get graphical images of your heart rate during your workout.

But most of all I love the instant readout that an HRM gives me on a particular organ in my body. I understand that all my organs benefit from exercise, but my HRM gives me a connection that is direct and fundamental.

To get cardiovascular benefit **you must increase your heart rate during exercise**. All of the exercise plans in this book are designed to get your heart rate up, and they frequently feature leg exercises followed by upper-body exercises to make your heart work harder by pumping blood from one end of your body to the other.

My exercise philosophy is one of intensity, whether you're in the weight room, the group-fitness studio, outside or even at home. This way you don't have to worry about the mix between cardio and strength training to benefit your heart, 'cos it's going to be pumping regardless!

HEART RATE TARGETS

Your maximum heart rate is calculated by subtracting your age from 220. For a moderately intense workout you should be training at around 50–70 per cent of your maximum heart rate (MHR), and for a vigorous training session around 70–85 per cent.

If fat loss is your goal, don't get sucked into the old 'fat burning range' of 65 per cent of your MHR. The faster your heart is beating, the more energy your body needs in a shorter period of time, so **go hard and amp it up**!

The two principal factors in improving your fitness are the length of your workout and the intensity at which you train.

JAYNE'S STORY

Soon after the birth of my third child, my daughter became sick with severe asthma. It was a tough time – in and out of hospital, my other two kids away from me, and my partner working a lot. I became depressed and turned to food for comfort.

Looking at some holiday photos there was one that just stood out to me. I was overweight and simply not happy in myself. I knew I had to find a way to change how I was feeling. I had had enough; I wanted to turn things around formyself and my family.

Michelle's program is like no other. It's so inspiring. It encouraged me to be active and eat healthily. It was just what I needed.

The 'getting active' part of the program was new to me. I had never been someone who loved sport, exercise or even enjoyed these things at school – they scared me and I always tried to get out of them. But I had to start somewhere. I started off with walks, then joined the gym, joined group classes and I soon found myself working out six days a week! I got used to it and loved it! I felt amazing. Exercise now gives me that time to myself, to work on myself mentally and physically so I can come back a better daughter, sister, mother and partner. I feel like I've regained my life – and lost 31 kilograms in the process! I went from a couch potato to an exercise addict. I now participate in all kind of events to challenge myself and meet with my friends at the local oval to workout together! I also feel that I have become a better role model for my children.

I didn't think it was possible when I started to be able to change my body so much after having three children close together. My goals are endless now! I now face my fears and have learnt that it's so liberating when I do.

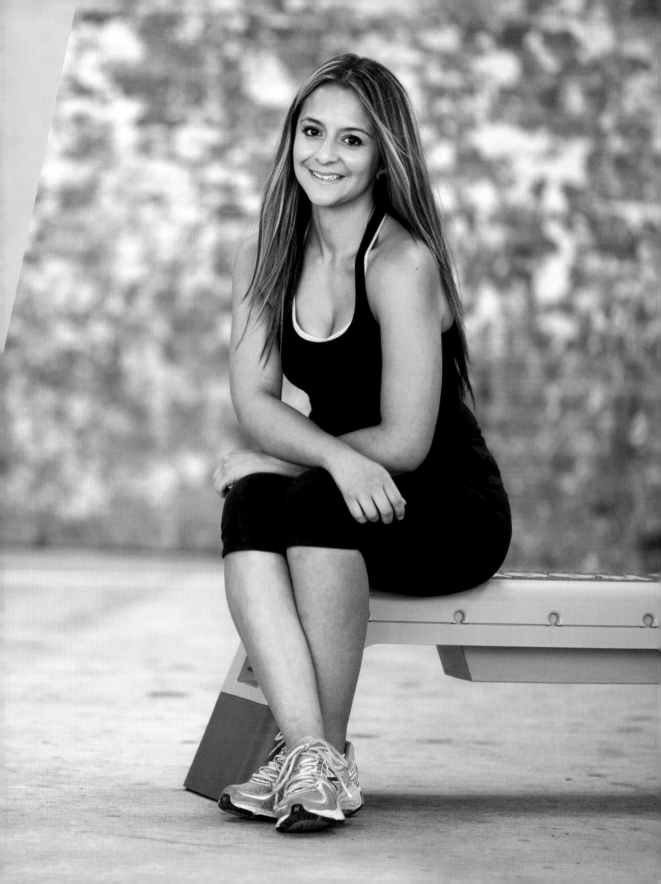

Okay, it's time to start working out. Step-by-step guides show you how to safely and effectively perform movements, before my two-week program delivers a slammin' training plan.

PLYOMETRICS /

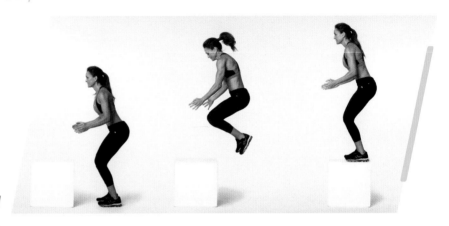

BOX JUMPS /

Use a bench or box for these. With your shoulders back and down, and your core pulled in, sink low into your legs, swing your arms back and launch upwards to land securely on top of the box. / Initially, step down, with a view to jumping down as you get more experienced. / Keep your knees and toes aligned at all times, with your legs acting as shock absorbers.

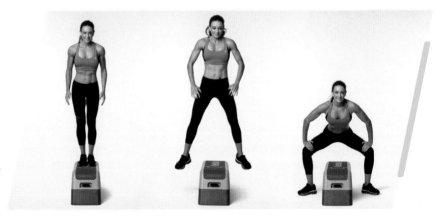

STRADDLE BOX JUMPS /

Stand on top of a step, with good posture, shoulders back and down, and your core pulled in. / Jump out with a wide stance and both knees angled outwards, with your toes following the same direction. / Brace through the core and land low placing your hands on your knees for support then spring immediately back to the starting position.

SQUAT JUMPS /

Start with your feet in a wide stance, with your heels slightly wider than your shoulders, toes and knees aligned and angled out, core pulled in, chest proud and hands linked behind your head, without pulling your head forward. / Sink deep into a squat then power up into a jump, maintaining the wide stance. / When you land, sink back into your starting position.

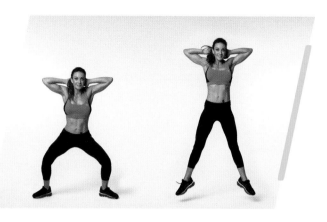

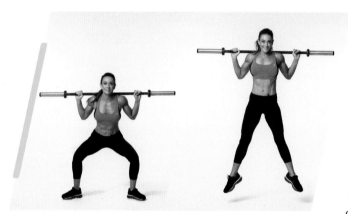

SQUAT JUMPS WITH A BAR

Place a metal weightlifting bar on the meaty part of your upper back and hold securely with a wide grip. / With your shoulders back and down, and core pulled in, place your heels shoulder-width apart with your toes and knees angled out in the same direction. / Brace through the core, bend into a squat and power up into a jump, landing softly and down into the initial squat position.

SKIPPING /

Using a skipping rope, jump with your legs acting as shock absorbers, maintaining knee and toe alignment and bracing your core. / Keep your hands out to the side, while your wrists need to work through a circular action to keep the rope moving.

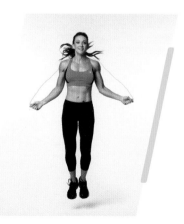

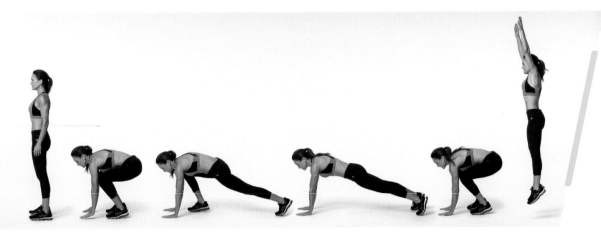

/ BURPEE (*beginner*)

From a standing position, crouch down and place your hands on the floor, either side of your feet. / Step one leg back and then follow with the other so you are in a 'plank' position. / Immediately step one foot in then the next, and as you stand up do a 'springboard' jump and clap your hands overhead.

/ BURPEE (*advanced*)

From a standing position, crouch down and place your hands on the floor, either side of your feet. / Brace through your core and jump both legs back, landing on your toes so you are in a 'plank' position with your legs straight. / Immediately jump both feet back in, and as you stand up do a 'springboard' jump and clap your hands overhead.

JUMPING CHIN-UPS /

Place a step underneath a pull-up bar. / Stand on the step and place your hands onto the bar, then use the spring from your legs to jump you up to a point where your chin is level with the bar. / This should be a continuous movement; however, rest if you have to, then get back to it.

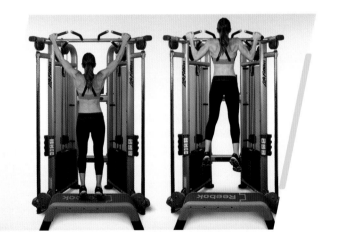

CARDIO /

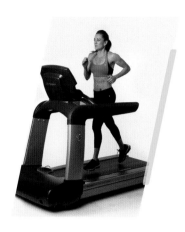

RUNNING /

This can be done either outdoors or on a treadmill. / With time you will pick up your speed, however, start with a mix of jogging and walking, gradually building up. / You will be surprised at how quickly your body adapts and can handle longer distances and quicker times if you put the work in.

/ CROSS TRAINER

The great thing about this piece of equipment is that you get a cardio workout similar to that of a run, without the impact on the legs. / You can use interval programs or work manually. / I will often use both high and medium intensity levels in approximately 30-second blocks. / I tend to work to my music – medium intensity in the verse, high intensity in the chorus!

ROWING MACHINE /

A 500-metre sprint on the rowing machine is a great way to kick off a workout once you are warmed up. / The idea with rowing is to do long smooth strokes, so aim to have the chain 'still', not bouncing around, and focus on long powerful strokes rather than short fast ones.

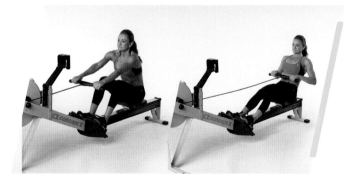

BOXING

Take a boxing class or work with a personal trainer who specialises in boxing to get some great advice about positioning, movement, and wrist and hand protection. / Boxing is one of my favourite ways to train. It's a great calorie-smasher, and I will often incorporate 2–3 minutes on the punch bag into my training sessions.

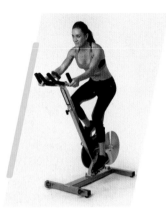

/ BIKE

Use upright bikes, preferably one where you can push out into sprints and hill climbs – spin bikes are the best for this. / Be sure your seat height is correct – when seated your foot at the lowest point on the pedal should have a slight bend in the knee (30 degrees or so). / Make sure the handles are in a position that allows you to maintain a relatively long straight back, and that your foot straps are secure. / Resistance is a must on these bikes; otherwise you are pedalling against fresh air!

The best workout programs combine cardio and weight training. Along with a healthy diet, it's the best way to exercise your body and its organs, boost your metabolism and lose weight.

LEGS /

TAP-DOWNS /

Start by standing tall on a bench with a dumbbell in each hand. / Lower one foot down to the floor only to barely touch the floor and come straight back up. / Maintain a long spine, shoulders back and down, chest proud, core pulled in and knee-toe alignment of the bent leg. / You naturally will lean forward at the bottom of this movement to maintain balance. / The movement should be fluid and constant.

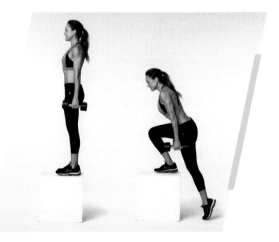

BULGARIAN SPLIT LUNGE /

With a dumbbell in each hand, place one foot up on a bench and position your grounded foot far enough away from the bench so you can lunge and maintain the position of the knee directly above the ankle. / Think 'north and south' throughout this movement, not 'east and west'. / Maintain strong posture throughout, as this will assist your balance.

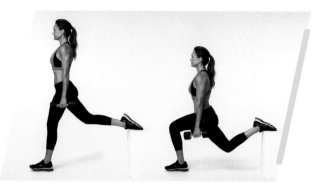

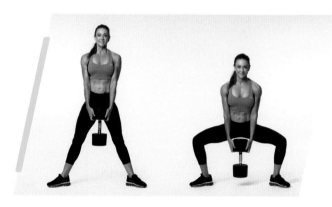

DUMBBELL SUMO SQUAT

Take a wide stance, toes and knees turned slightly outward and aligned. / Squat down until the dumbbell almost touches the ground then stand back up. / Maintain a strong posture, with chest proud, shoulders back and down, and core pulled in.

OVERHEAD BARBELL WALKING LUNGES /

Using a wide grip, hold a barbell directly overhead. / Stand with your feet hip-width apart and pull your core in. / Step forward and sink into a lunge whereby the front knee remains directly above the ankle, not forward of it. In the lunge, both legs should be bent at a right angle. / Push back up, bringing your back leg forward, into the initial stance. / You must maintain a tall long posture without bending forward through the torso. / Focus on pushing the barbell up towards the roof and away from you.

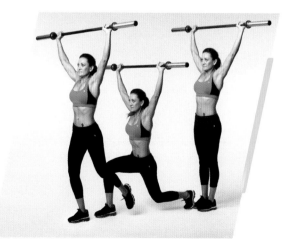

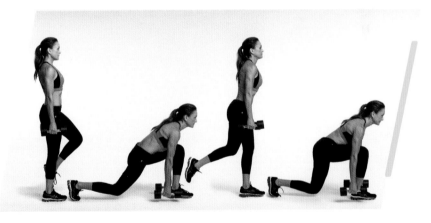

DUMBBELL LUNGE/ SQUAT/ LUNGE/ SQUAT JUMP /

This is a sequence of four movements joined together to make a great leg training exercise. / With feet shoulder-width apart, step forward with your right leg into a lunge then back. / Perform a squat, then step the left leg forward into a lunge, coming back to perform a squat with a jump. / As you move through the sequence the jumps will go up by one until you reach five in a row. / Of course, you can go to any number you wish and you can also start with the higher number of jumps and bring them down one by one.

WALKING LUNGE WITH A LOW REACH /

These lunges attack not only the legs, but open the glutes right up, while also bringing the back into play. / They take time to perfect, so build your weights up gradually. / With a dumbbell in each hand, stand with your feet hip-width apart. / Step forward and long into a walking lunge while bending down, maintaining strong posture, to touch the dumbbells either side of the foot. / Then come up into standing position and repeat on the other side. / Be sure to keep your back straight during the bend over.

BACK /

BENT-OVER ROWS WITH DUMBBELLS /

Holding dumbbells in each hand, stand with your feet hip-width apart. / With your knees bent, bend over, maintaining a long straight back and proud chest as your hands hang below your shoulders. / Now pull the dumbbells up into your hips, keeping your elbows tucked in. Your torso will also move upward, but never to fully upright. / Feel the pinch between your shoulderblades.

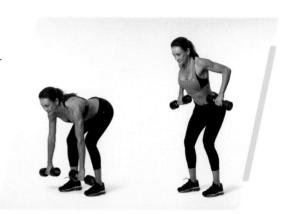

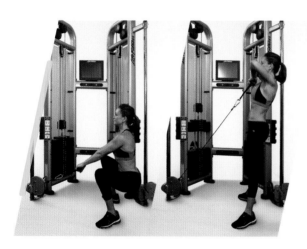

/ CABLE ROW WITH SQUAT

Using a heavy weight on the cable machine and a low positioned cable, step back from the machine with a shoulder-width stance. / Squat down low, maintaining a long upright straight back, with arms extended forward. / Now push up on your feet, pulling the cable handles towards your lower rib cage, and squeezing between the shoulder blades.

DEADLIFTS /

Using a barbell with weights, stand tall, feet hip-width apart, core pulled in, shoulders back and down, and chest proud. / Slide the barbell down your legs while maintaining a long straight spine. / You will need to bend at the knees, push your butt back and lift your tailbone to assist with posture. / The barbell may just touch the floor or get to within an inch or two (depending on the flexibility in your hamstrings). / Return to the starting position.

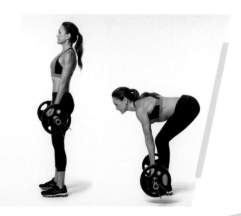

ONE-ARM ROW WITH OPPOSITE LEG EXTENSION

In one hand hold a dumbbell or kettle bell. / Place your other hand on a bench or box for support and extend the leg on the same side long and behind. / The dumbbell or kettle bell should now hang directly below the shoulder. Pull it up into the hip while rotating or 'rolling' the body. / Try to keep everything still and balanced by pulling in the core and holding your body tight.

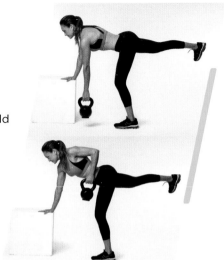

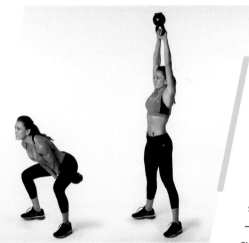

KETTLE-BELL SWINGS

Stand with feet shoulder-width apart, with toes and knees slightly angled out and the kettle bell on the floor. / Grab the kettle bell with both hands and begin to swing, maintaining a long spine, with chest proud, and shoulders back and down. / The kettle bell should move directly between your legs, and your forearms should touch the inside of your thighs. / Use an explosive drive from your legs, squeezing your butt, to swing the bell forward – it all comes from below the waist. Begin by swinging the bell to chest height. / Once you are feeling confident, you can take it to the next level by swinging higher, as shown in the picture. / Be sure that the bell is always slightly angled forward so it doesn't go too far behind your head and you lose balance or drop it.

Don't go too hard, too fast. That way you're more likely to injure yourself or get demotivated. Gradually up the time and intensity of your workouts and you'll be much more likely to stick with it.

64

CHEST /

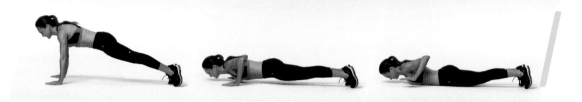

/ PUSH-UPS

Start in an upright push-up position, with a long torso like a plank of wood, core pulled in, with shoulders back and down away from your ears. / Lower yourself down to an inch off the floor then push yourself back up. / Maintain a strong body throughout, with no bending or arching through the middle line.

/ HAND RELEASE PUSH-UPS

These are very similar to regular push-ups, however you will actually lie down and release your hands off the floor by approximately an inch. / All the same principles apply with regards to body alignment. / The difference is you know you are working through a full range of movement. / Neither is better than the other, they are simply two different ways to train. I use both.

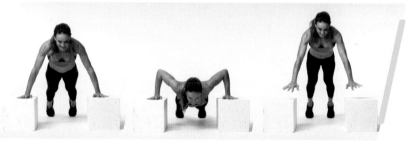

PLYOMETRIC PUSH-UPS

Set yourself up between two benches or boxes with enough room for your body to move easily. / The same principles of body alignment apply as with any other push-up, however, from the bottom of this push-up you must explode up so your hands jump from the benches. / Land softly and repeat the movement. / Don't go too deep in the down phase; chest level or slightly lower than the bench is far enough.

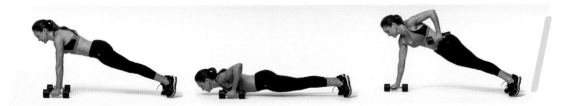

MAN-MAKER ROWS /

Holding two light to medium dumbbells, assume a push-up position. / Lower yourself down and as you push up, pull one hand into the hip without too much rotation through the body. / Lower your hand down, go back down into the push-up and repeat on the other side.

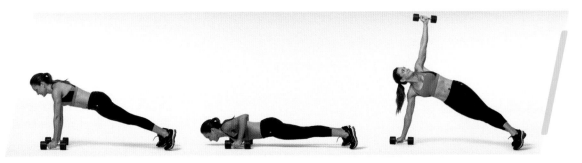

MAN-MAKER PRESS /

This is an advanced variation on the above whereby, instead of pulling the dumbbell into the hip, you pull it up towards the chest, twist through the torso and continue to press from the shoulder up to the roof. / Be sure you feel a strong push upwards from the stationary shoulder below, as this is your support foundation. / Good luck – these hurt!

SHOULDERS /

STANDING DUMBBELL PRESS /

Start with your feet hip-width apart, knees slightly bent and leg muscles holding strong. / Hold a dumbbell in each hand, positioned level with your chin and slightly forward of your shoulders. / Press both hands up simultaneously until your arms are fully extended. / Keep your core pulled in, chest proud, and your shoulders back and down.

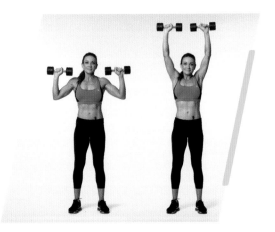

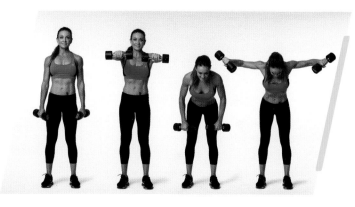

FRONT RAISE WITH BENT-OVER FLY

This combines two movements in one. Holding a light to medium dumbbell in each hand, stand tall with chest proud, shoulders back and down, and core pulled in. / Brace your body as you raise both dumbbells out in front, with your elbows turned slightly outward, then lower down while simultaneously lowering your body forward by bending the knees and pushing your butt back. / Maintain a straight back by lifting your tailbone up and pushing your chest out. / Now raise the dumbbells out to the side, level with your shoulders. / Aim to point your elbows to the back, arms slightly bent. / Stand up and repeat.

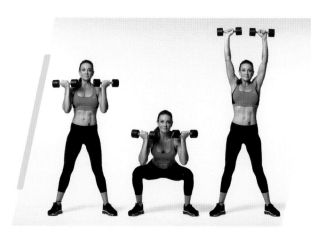

ARNOLD PRESS WITH SQUAT

Start with your feet shoulder-width apart, toes and knees slightly angled out. / With your core pulled in, chest proud, and shoulders back and down, place the dumbbells level with your chin with palms facing in. / Be sure that the dumbbells are not 'resting' on your chest. / Squat down into a low squat, maintaining perfect posture, then explode up into a shoulder press where the dumbbells will fluidly turn ending with your palms facing forward at the top of the press.

Grouping exercises together and adding variations is a good way of engaging a wider range of muscles and keeping your workouts interesting.

DUMBBELL SQUAT PRESS /

Start with your feet approximately shoulder-width apart, or slightly closer, depending on how the movement feels as you go down. / Pull your core in and squat down into a low squat position while bending forward to bring your dumbbells close to the floor on either side of your legs. / It's important to maintain strong posture (chest up, shoulders back), so note how far down you can go before you lose your posture. / Drive up strong through the legs as you bring the dumbbells to your shoulders, and then power them up into a shoulder press.

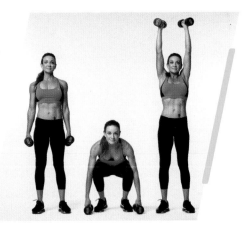

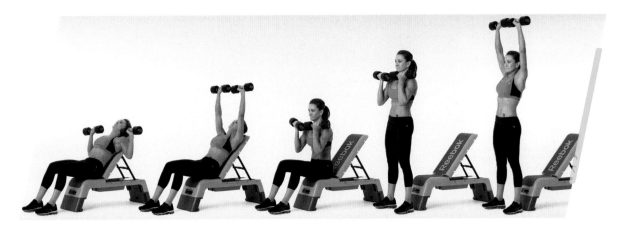

MISHY MAKER /

Lie down on an incline bench, feet shoulder width apart and flat on the floor, and hold the weights by your shoulders. / Perform a bench press, lifting the weights straight out from your shoulders until your arms are straight but not locked. / Slowly bring the weights back into your body while at the same time rising to a sitting position. / Keeping the weights by your shoulders, stand up. / Raise the weights above you, until your arms are straight but not locked. / Slowly lower the weights back towards your shoulders. / Try to move through the stages as fluidly as possible.

Squat presses are a prime example of a super compound exercise because they engage your arms, core, shoulders and legs. They rock!

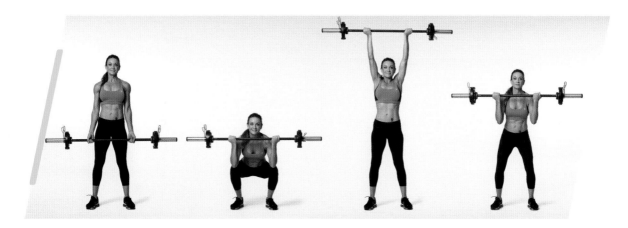

BICEP CURL SQUAT PRESS

This is another variation giving you more mileage from this awesome move. / Using a barbell with weight, start with perfect posture, core pulled in, chest proud and shoulders back and down. / Then sink down into a squat while simultaneously curling the barbell up. / Maintain strong posture with shoulders back and core pulled in as you powerfully drive up, pressing the barbell overhead. / Bring the bar down to your chest then curl down into the start position and repeat.

MEDICINE BALL PRESS

Yet another version of the press, this time using a medium to heavy medicine ball. / Start with your feet shoulder-width apart, toes and knees slightly turned out, and holding the ball. / Squat down low with the ball held at chest level then drive up powerfully from the legs, throwing the ball up into the air. / As you catch the ball, start to sink back down into the squat so it's all one fluid movement. / In the picture I have a box to tap my butt on each time so I know I go full depth. / You can also mark a height on a wall and try to get the ball up to that height every throw.

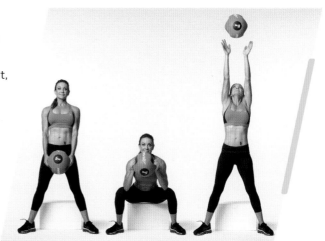

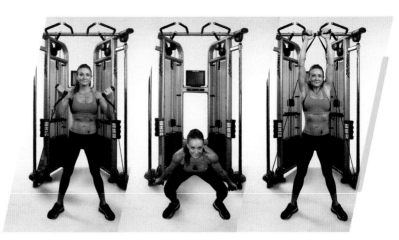

CABLE SHOULDER PRESS WITH SQUAT

Cables add an extra 'zing' to this movement as the tension is 'on' throughout. / Start with a cable handle in each hand and, depending on the cable machine, position yourself so you will have tension throughout the move. / Place your feet shoulder-width apart, with toes and knees slightly angled out. / Bend down into a squat. / Due to the cables you will need to lean forward in this movement, however keep your chest up, your shoulders back and your core pulled in. / Drive up through the legs and powerfully press the cables up over your head. / This one takes some practice, so start with a light weight.

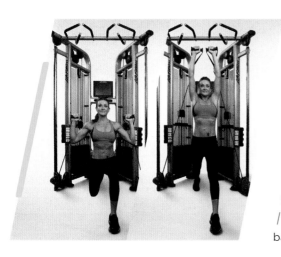

CABLE SHOULDER PRESS WITH LUNGE

Holding the cable handles, position yourself squarely between them and so you can take a long lunge position, allowing the front knee to remain directly above the ankle, not shoot forward over it. / At the bottom of the lunge, both legs should be at a right angle. / Start with the cable handles at shoulder height, lower down into the lunge and drive up with a shoulder press. / You will need to pull your core in, not only for back support but also for balance assistance.

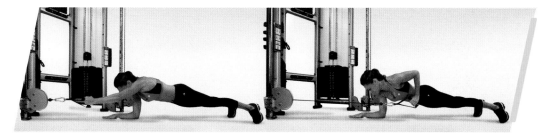

PLANK CABLE ROW /

Grab the cable and slide yourself back away from the cable machine so that with your arm fully extended in front of you there is still tension on the cable. / From there position yourself into a plank, with one arm extended. / Try to maintain level hips, a strong torso and legs to maintain a still body through out the movement. / Draw your abs up toward the ceiling and lock into position to assist this. / Breath out as you pull the cable back toward your hip, breathe in as you release.

Don't think your training isn't making a difference to your body and mind. Your cells respond the moment you do the first rep, or take the first steps of a run.

CORE /

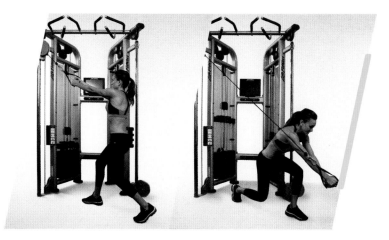

CABLE WOODCHOPS /

Take the cable setting up to the highest point and use only one handle for both hands. / Position your legs in a half lunge and face the cable. / Maintain strong straight arms; do not bend them through the movement as you cut through the air, taking a line the furthest distance away from you. It all comes from the core, so brace, and pivot your body down through a diagonal movement finishing in a half lunge, hand pointing towards the floor. / Control the movement on the way up; power it on the way down.

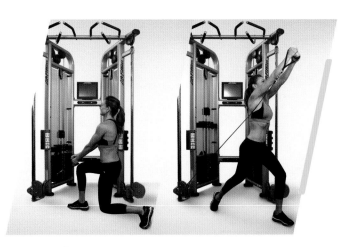

CABLE DISCUS THROW /

This is the exact opposite of the cable woodchops. / Take the cable setting down to the lowest point. / Start in a lunge position with a long spine and hands down near your ankles. / Drive up, using your core and legs, cutting a diagonal line the furthest distance away from you. / Maintain strong straight arms. / There should not be too much leaning forward with the body in the lowest point; instead bend and use your legs. / Imagine you are hurling that discus at the Olympics! / Control the movement on the downward phase.

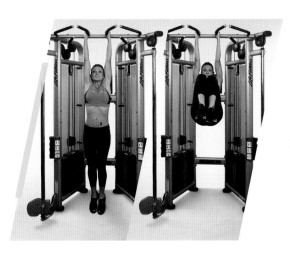

/ HANGMAN

Holding on to a chin-up bar or any secure bar, drive your knees up together and try to touch your chest or get as close as possible. / Then lower your legs. / Use control to avoid too much swinging. / For a variation, add a twist and bring your knees towards one of your armpits.

Pay as much attention to your diet as you do to your training. Each nutritious, wholefood meal is like a well-planned, well-executed workout.

STRETCHING /

DOWNWARD DOG /

Start on your hands and knees. / Spread your fingers. / Exhale and lift your knees from the floor, pushing your tailbone towards the ceiling. / Push your thighs back and stretch your heels towards the floor. / Straighten your knees without a full 'lockout'. / Hold for 30-60 seconds, rest back on knees the then go again. / Do this stretch at least three times.

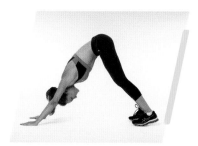

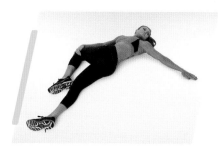

/ BACK TWIST

Lying on your back bring your right knee up into your chest then using the left hand to knee, drag the knee across your body. / Take your right arm, extend it out long to the side of you and look down the length of that arm. / Breath deeply, then as you exhale 'sink' deeper into the stretch. / Hold the stretch for 30-60 seconds then repeat on the other side. / Do both sides at least twice.

SITTING GLUTE /

Sit with your arms behind you propping you up, both knees bent. / Cross one leg over the other, bent leg. The knee should point directly out to the side. / Now 'lift' up through your chest, focusing on strong posture. Pull your shoulders back and down and lengthen your spine, then bring your 'proud' chest forward toward the inside of your ankle. / Hold this stretch for 30-60 seconds then swap. / Do this stretch as least twice on both sides.

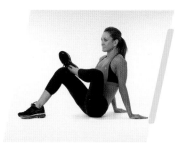

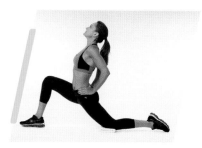

/ HIP FLEXOR

In a kneeling lunge position, place a folded towel under the knee for comfort. Position the back leg long behind you and the front leg in a right angle. / Place your hands on your hips, to encourage a proud chest, and focus on your posture, with shoulders back, and a long spine. / Breathe deeply and 'sink' down towards the floor. / Hold for 30-60 seconds then swap. / Repeat at least twice on each side.

QUADS AGAINST THE WALL /

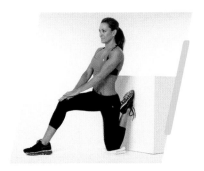

With your back against a wall, crouch down. / Fold one leg up against the wall and place a rolled up towel under your knee for comfort. / Have the other leg positioned in a right angle in front and place your hands to that leg for support while lifting up through your torso, focusing on perfect posture, drawing you core inwards and lifting the chest. / Move your body back toward the wall to gain a deeper stretch, breathe deeply and gently work through this stretch, holding for 30–60 seconds before swapping to the other side. / Repeat this stretch at least twice on both sides.

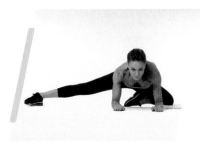

/ INNER THIGH

Place a folded towel on the floor and kneel down your left knee on the towel. / Lean forward so that your forearms are flat on the floor with your palms down. / Stretch your right leg out to the side, keeping it straight. / Bring your left foot forward so it is under your bottom. / Try to keep the toes of the extended leg pointing forward. / Hold for 15–20 seconds then repeat on the other side.

CHEST /

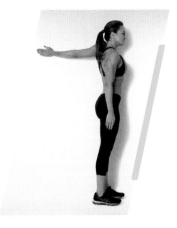

Stand side on to a wall and place the closest hand onto the wall so that it is palm down and the arm is straight out behind you. / Focus on perfect posture, draw the core in, lift up through the chest and draw your shoulders back and down. / Start to turn your body away from the wall. / You will feel a stretch running across one side of your chest, the front of your shoulder and along your bicep. Hold for 30–60 seconds, then swap. / Repeat two or three times on both sides.

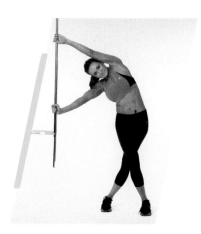

/ SIDE HOLDING BAR

Using a solid bar or piece of equipment in the gym, stand beside the bar and reach over with a shoulder width grip. / Tuck the leg furthest away from the bar behind you, keeping your hips square on. / Maintain a long spine and core pulled in as you push your hips out to the side, slightly pulling against the bar. Avoid twisting the body. / You should feel the stretch run entirely down one side including the leg. / Hold for 30–60 seconds then swap. / Repeat at least twice through on each side.

SHOULDER MOBILITY /

Hold a lightweight bar or broom stick with a wide grip. / Gradually work the bar over your head and to behind your back. / Stand tall with your shoulders pulled back and down. Keep a long spine, chest proud, and core pulled in. / It may take some weeks before you can work that bar through the full range of movement. Don't force it. Work it slowly and take your time.

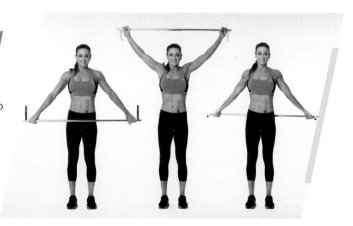

/ CALF OFF A STEP

You see me doing these anytime I am on an escalator or standing chatting if there is a step around. / Place one heel off the edge of a step and drop your weight straight down into that heel. / Start with a straight leg and then after around 30 seconds, bend the knee, keeping it aligned with the toes. You will feel the stretch change and move lower into the back of the ankle. / Hold for another 30 seconds then swap legs. / Repeat two or three times on each side.

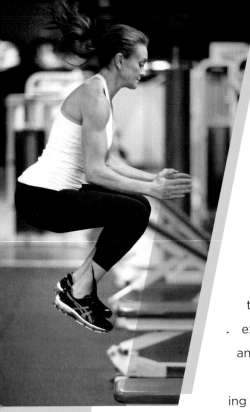

YOUR BEST BODY CIRCUITS /

All the workouts in *Your Best Body* are designed to help you achieve just that – the best version of you in terms of overall fitness, strength, coordination, mobility and agility.

However, **you can shift the emphasis of your workouts for specific goals.** If, for instance, I am tuning myself up for a running event, then I will steer the ship more towards high-end fitness or cardio exercises. If I am training for an obstacle course, then I will specifically select exercises that are strength-based, increasing the weight and lowering the number of reps.

Generally, I like to mix up my workouts to avoid becoming bored and complacent.

WARM-UP

Your warm-up is non-negotiable. It's important both physically and mentally that you warm your body up before you start any training. Spend approximately 10 minutes warming yourself up by mixing the different modalities listed below. It's smart to know what you will be doing in your circuit and to choose a warm-up that directly targets those muscle groups.

Warm-up modalities:

- 5 minutes on cross trainer
- 5 minutes on treadmill
- 5 minutes on rowing machine
- 5 minutes skipping
- 5 minutes light outdoor jog (heels up, knees up)
- 5 minutes on a set of stairs
- 5 minutes mixing squats, push-ups, step-ups and lunges.

CIRCUITS

You will see when you get to my week one and week two schedules that you can utilise a wide variety of exercises to mix up your training and keep your body guessing. Here are some variables to show you how you can create **different workouts for different outcomes** to your training, keeping it exciting and stopping you getting bored. Please don't be limited by them though; there are a gazillion more combinations you can put together.

Choose the Circuit

- A mixed bag of fitness, strength, upper and lower body plus plyometric movements
- Predominately strength based for upper and/or lower body
- All-out fitness assault with plenty of multiple muscle groups working
- Strength and fitness based with a focus on legs
- Strength and fitness based with a focus on upper body.

Choose the Weight

- 100 per cent of your maximum weight with very low repetitions (3–5).
- 50–70 per cent of your maximum with medium repetitions (8–12).
- 20–40 per cent of your maximum with high repetitions (15–50).
- No weight – many exercises are simply body weight and will often be high in repetition.

As a personal trainer, I know that it's impossible to do a 'one size fits all' with weights. One of my girlfriends, for example, weighs only 48 kilos but is as strong as a bull! You will very quickly learn what feels too light or too heavy – **your body will tell you where you're at**. But you will need to 'man up' as well, so no goofing off and going too light. My technique usually gets a little messy by the last few repetitions, but that's a good sign – if I'm not heaving by the last few reps, then I know its time to increase the weight.

CHOOSE THE REPS

- Keep in mind that high-weight, low-repetition exercises will be more strength based. The high-repetition, low-weight exercises will be fitness based.
- You can go from as few as three repetitions to as high as 50 repetitions depending on the weight. Mixing different numbers of reps into one circuit is a good idea.

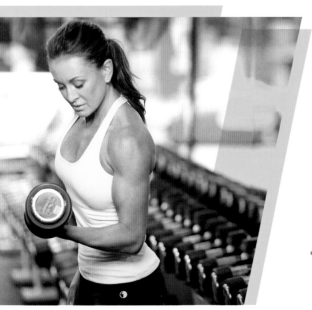

CHOOSE THE TIME

- Complete as many rounds of the circuit as you can in 20 minutes. Rest where you have to, but try to keep on the move.
- Do as many rounds of the circuit in three minutes, rest for one minute and repeat a further four more times, trying to complete more rounds in the given three minutes (5 x 3-minute rounds total).
- Time yourself for you first round of the circuit. Try to beat that time for round two and possibly round three.

There are no rules about how you set up your circuit, so be creative! Keep in mind, however, what your focus and desired outcome is.

There is ONE GOLDEN RULE to stick to.

Always make a plan BEFORE you get to the gym, and then NAIL IT!

Keep a logbook of your circuits, weights, repetitions and times. This is a highly motivating and valuable tool to benchmark yourself and chart your improvement. Always leave it in your gym bag.

Logbook example

mixed weights and reps circuit	rounds
• 5 x bent-over rows with barbell (heavy weight)	
• 30 x box jumps	
• 10 x plyometric push-ups	
• 20 x walking lunges with a low reach (medium to heavy dumbbells)	

Do as many rounds as you can in 20 mins

top-end fitness or cardio circuit	rounds
• Run 400 metres	
• 20 x squat jump with bar (medium weight bar)	
• 20 x tap-downs, 10 each leg (medium to light weight)	
• 20 x box jumps	
• 20 x push-ups	

Do as many rounds as you can in 25 mins

pyramid training with your repetitions	rounds
• 30 x barbell walking lunges	
• 30 x kettle-bell swings	
• 30 x medicine-ball shoulder press with squat	
• 16 x barbell walking lunges	
• 16 x kettle-bell swings	
• 16 x medicine-ball shoulder press with squat	
• 8 x barbell walking lunges	
• 8 x kettle-bell swings	
• 8 x medicine-ball shoulder press with squat	

If you're up to it, work through the pyramid in reverse, increasing the reps. Decrease the weight if you need to

YOUR BEST STANDARD CIRCUITS /

Here are some really simple stock standard circuits. Mostly all I've said is do 20 reps of everything, and do five rounds, resting for no more than 1–2 minutes after each round. Because the repetitions are high, the weight should be light to medium (20–40 per cent of your maximum weight). If you're new to this kind of training, reduce the reps to 10 and build up from there.

When you first start out you may be only able to do two or three rounds of these circuits, so if you've never trained like this before, PLEASE don't feel that you have to do as many rounds as I have prescribed. As your fitness improves you will build up to four or five rounds. It took me a while to build up to five rounds, and some days I don't crack it.

These standards are great for when you don't want to think too much. So, what are you waiting for? Go!

Circuit 1		
1. 20 x straddle box jumps	4. 20 x Bulgarian split lunge (right leg back)
2. 10 x man-maker rows	5. Skip for 1 minute
3. 20 x Bulgarian split lunge (left leg back)	6. 20 x standing dumbbell press

Circuit 2		
1. 20 x walking lunge with low reach	4. 20 x hand release push-ups
2. 20 x jumping chin-ups	5. 20 x cable woodchops (both sides)
3. 20 x cable upright row with squat	6. 20 x front raise with bent-over fly

Circuit 3		
1. Treadmill run 400 metres as fast as you can	4. 20 x tap-downs (10 each leg)
2. 20 x medicine ball throw with squat	5. 20 x Arnold press with squat
3. 20 x bent-over dumbbell rows	6. 20 x plank cable pull (10 on each arm without dropping)

Circuit 4	1. 10 x burpees	4. 20 x dumbbell sumo squat
	2. 20 x deadlifts	5. 20 x cable woodchops (right side)
	3. 20 x cable shoulder press with lunge (10 each leg)	6. 20 x cable woodchops (left side)

YOUR BEST LEGS AND BUTT CIRCUITS /

Circuit 1	1. Treadmill run 400 metres as fast as you can	4. 20 x Bulgarian split lunges (20 each leg)
	2. 20 x squat jumps with or without a barbell	5. 20 x Arnold press with squat
	3. 20 x overhead barbell walking lunges	6. 20 x dumbbell sumo squat

Circuit 2	1. 20 x box jumps	4. 20 x walking lunges with a low reach
	2. 20 x cable shoulder press with squat	5. 1 x pyramid dumbbell sequence (see page 82: Tuesday)
	3. 20 x tap-downs (10 each leg)	

YOUR BEST UPPER BODY CIRCUITS /

Circuit 1	1. 20 x jumping chin-ups	4. 20 x one arm rows with opposite leg extension (10 each side)
	2. 10 x man makers, rows or press (5 each side, alternating)	5. 20 x push-ups
	3. 20 x bicep curl squat press	6. 20 x plank cable rows (10 each side)

Circuit 2	1. Skip for 1 minute	4. 20 x cable discus throw (left side)
	2. 20 x bent-over rows with dumbbell	5. 20 x hangman knees to chest
	3. 20 x cable discus throw (right side)	6. 20 x dumbbell squat with shoulder press

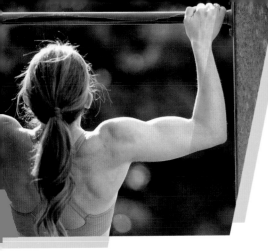

*Are you ready? Then let's go!
With these workouts you're
gonna feel amazing.
Promise!*

TWO-WEEK EXERCISE PROGRAM

Two weeks. Twelve days of exercises. Varied, fun workouts and a full-body training regime.

WEEK ONE

MONDAY / *Circuit focus: overall body strength and fitness*

Warm-up 10 minutes	Do four rounds, with minimal rest between rounds.	Full body stretch
	• 10 x burpees (normal or modified) • 20 x Bulgarian split lunge with dumbbells (medium to heavy) (10 each leg) • 15 x kettle-bell swings (medium to heavy) • 15 x jumping chin-ups • 15 x straddle box jumps • 10 x hangman (knees to chest)	
	Final Blast: 2 km run on treadmill	

TUESDAY / *Circuit focus: fitness and leg strength*

Warm-up 10 minutes	Do four rounds of this circuit, with rounds two and four reversing the pyramid sequence, working from five squat jumps down to one.	Full body stretch
	• Pyramid dumbbell sequence (medium weight) lunge/squat/lunge/ 1 x squat jump lunge/squat/lunge/ 2 x squat jump lunge/squat/lunge/ 3 x squat jump lunge/squat/lunge/ 4 x squat jump lunge/squat/lunge/ 5 x squat jump • 15 x bicep curl squat press (medium weight) • 16 x walking lunges with a low reach (medium weight) • 15 x Arnold press with squat (light to medium weight) • 10 x squat jumps	
	Final Blast: 20 x plank cable pull (10 on each arm) three times through (light weight)	

82

WEDNESDAY / *Circuit focus: fitness, agility and balance*

Warm-up 10 minutes

Do three to five rounds in total, time yourself for each round, 1–2 minutes rest, repeat. Aim to beat your first round time at least twice.

- Run 400 metres
- 20 x box jumps
- 30 x one arm row opposite leg extension (15 each side) (light to medium weight)
- 20 x squat jumps with a bar
- 15 x jumping chin-ups

Final Blast: 15 x hangman (knees to chest), three times through. Add some twisting for variation.

Full body stretch

THURSDAY / *Circuit focus: upper body strength and fitness*

Warm-up 10 minutes

Do this circuit with urgency, but maintaining form. Rest for 1–2 minutes after each round. Complete three to five rounds.

- 20 x bent-over rows with barbell (medium weight)
- 15 x mishy makers (medium weight)
- 10 x plyometric push-ups
- 10 x man-maker press (light–medium weight) (5 each side)
- Skip for 2 minutes flat out

Final Blast: indoor or outdoor jog or cross trainer for 10–15 minutes

Full body stretch

FRIDAY / *Circuit focus: core strength and fitness*

Warm-up 10 minutes

5 rounds in total. Each round gets progressively heavier but the reps go down.

- 30 x cable discus throw right (light weight)
- 30 x cable discus throw left (light weight)
- 30 x plank cable row (15 each arm) (light weight)
- 30 x cable woodchops right (light weight)
- 30 x cable woodchops left (light weight)
- 12 x hangman (no weight so these stay the same for each round)

Round 2: the reps go down to 20 and the weight comes up by 10 per cent

Round 3: the reps go down to 15 and the weight comes up by 10 per cent

Round 4: the reps go down to 10 and the weight comes up by 10 per cent

Round 5: the reps go down to 8 and weight is as heavy as you can handle

Full body stretch

By focusing on different areas of the body on different days, you get a complete workout and, importantly, won't get bored doing the same things all the time.

SATURDAY / *Circuit focus: everything! ALL OUT WAR!*

Go as hard as you possibly can within each round.
Rest 2–3 minutes between each circuit

Warm-up 10 minutes

Round 1
- 500-metre rowing machine sprint
- 30 x medicine-ball press (light to medium ball)
- 40 x tap-downs (20 each leg) (light to medium weight)
- 20 x cable shoulder press with squat (light to medium weight)
- 20 x cable woodchops right (light to medium weight)
- 20 x cable woodchops left (light to medium weight)
- 20 x box jumps

Round 2
- 300-metre rowing machine sprint
- 20 x medicine-ball press (slightly heavier weight)
- 30 x tap-downs (15 each leg) (slightly heavier weight)
- 15 x cable shoulder press squat (slightly heavier weight)
- 15 x cable woodchops right (slightly heavier weight)
- 15 x cable woodchops left (slightly heavier weight)
- 15 x box jumps

Round 3
- 200-metre rowing machine sprint
- 15 x medicine-ball press (slightly heavier weight)
- 20 x tap-downs (10 each leg) (slightly heavier weight)
- 10 x cable shoulder press with squat (slightly heavier weight)
- 10 x cable woodchops right (slightly heavier weight)
- 10 x cable woodchops left (slightly heavier weight)
- 10 x box jumps

Final Blast: Repeat Round 1, only reducing the weights if you have to

Full body stretch

SUNDAY / *Rest*

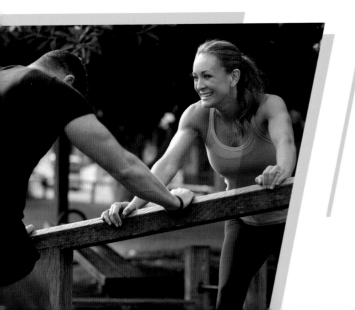

Stretching after a workout is essential, so don't blow it off even if you are in a hurry. It prevents soreness, helps increase flexibility and guards against injury.

WEEK TWO

MONDAY / *Circuit focus: overall body strength and fitness.*

Warm-up 10 minutes

Today I have given you two smaller circuits. Do the first one three times with a two-minute rest between each round, then head to the next circuit and do the same.

Round 1
- 20 x cable upright row with squat (light to medium weight)
- 20 x squat jumps
- 20 x cable shoulder press with lunge (10 each leg) (light to medium weight)

Round 2
- 15 x jumping chin-ups
- 20 x straddle box jumps
- 15 x mishy makers (light to medium weight)

Final Blast: 20 x plank cable row (10 each side) twice through (medium weight)

Full body stretch

TUESDAY / *Circuit focus: fitness and leg strength*

Warm-up 10 minutes

Do four rounds. Start with light weights and high reps, building up each round with heavier weight but less reps. Rest for two minutes between rounds

- 30 x overhead barbell walking lunges (light weight)
- 30 x dumbbell sumo squats (light weight)
- 30 x Bulgarian split lunges (15 each leg) (light weight)
- Skip for 2 minutes (this will remain the same throughout)
- 30 x kettle-bell swings (light weight)
- 30 x straddle box jumps (no weight)

Round 2: the reps go down to 20 and the weight comes up by 10 per cent

Round 3: the reps go down to 15 and the weight comes up by 10 per cent

Round 4: the reps go down to 10 and weight is as heavy as you can handle

Final Blast: 5 minutes of jogging

Full body stretch

WEDNESDAY / *Circuit focus: fitness, agility and balance*

Warm-up 10 minutes

Today the focus is on how long the overall session takes you. I'd like you to aim for five rounds but see how you go. Give yourself a time limit of say 35 minutes to complete the whole thing. Regardless of how long it takes, you now have a benchmark to try to beat next time.

- 10 x burpees (normal or modified)
- 20 x Arnold press with squat (light to medium weight)
- 20 x one-arm row with opposite leg extension (10 each side) (light to medium weight)
- 15 x box jumps
- 10 x man maker rows (5 each side) (light to medium weight)
- 10 x bicep curl squat press (light to medium weight)

Final Blast: 15 x hangman, three times through (add some twisting for variation)

Full body stretch

THURSDAY / *Circuit focus: upper body and fitness*

Focus on selecting a weight that will have you only just getting to 15 reps. Try having two sets of weights, a heavier set and a lighter set. Start with the heavy and only move to the light if you can't finish the reps. Do 4 to 5 rounds with a sense of urgency, but maintaining form.

- 15 x bent-over rows with dumbbells (medium weight)
- 15 x mishy makers (medium weight)
- 15 x medicine-ball press (medium weight)
- 12 x man-maker press (6 each side) (light to medium weight)
- 15 x jumping chin-ups

Final Blast: hit the cross trainer for 5 minutes, going hard

Warm-up 10 minutes

Full body stretch

FRIDAY / *Circuit focus – core strength and fitness*

Today you have three circuits of only two exercises. Move quickly and do each round three times through before moving onto the next.

Round 1
- 30 x cable woodchops (15 each side) (light weight, building up each round)
- 30 x cable discus throw (15 each side) (light weight, building up each round)

Round 2
- 15 x cable shoulder press with squat (light weight, building up each round)
- 20 x plank cable row (10 each side) (light weight, building up each round)

Round 3
- 15 x box jumps
- 15 x hand release push-ups

Final Blast: 1 km sprint on treadmill, fast!

Warm-up 10 minutes

Full body stretch

SATURDAY / *Circuit focus: WORLD DOMINATION!*

Okay, this one is gonna hurt, so how many rounds? As many as you can in 40 minutes, running between each station. It's a long time, so if you have to pause keep it to 30 seconds or so before continuing. Good luck, sunshine!

- 500 m sprint on rowing machine (medium resistance)
- 40 x kettle-bell swings (medium to heavy weight)
- 10 x burpees (normal or modified)
- 20 x walking lunges with a low reach (medium to heavy weight)
- 15 x squat jumps with a bar
- 20 x cable shoulder press with squat (medium weight)

Final Blast: 30 x hangman

Warm-up 10 minutes

Full body stretch

SUNDAY / *Rest*

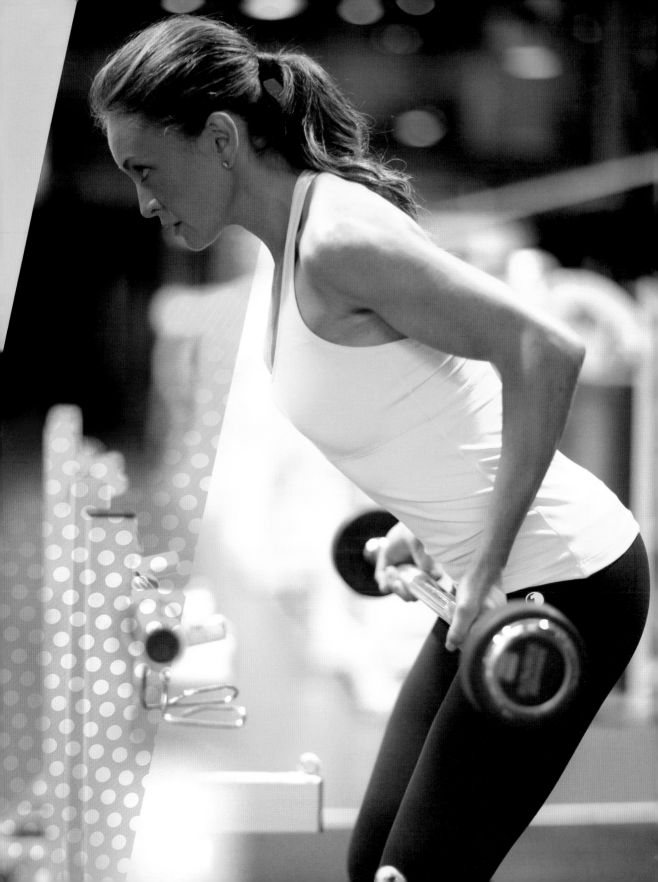

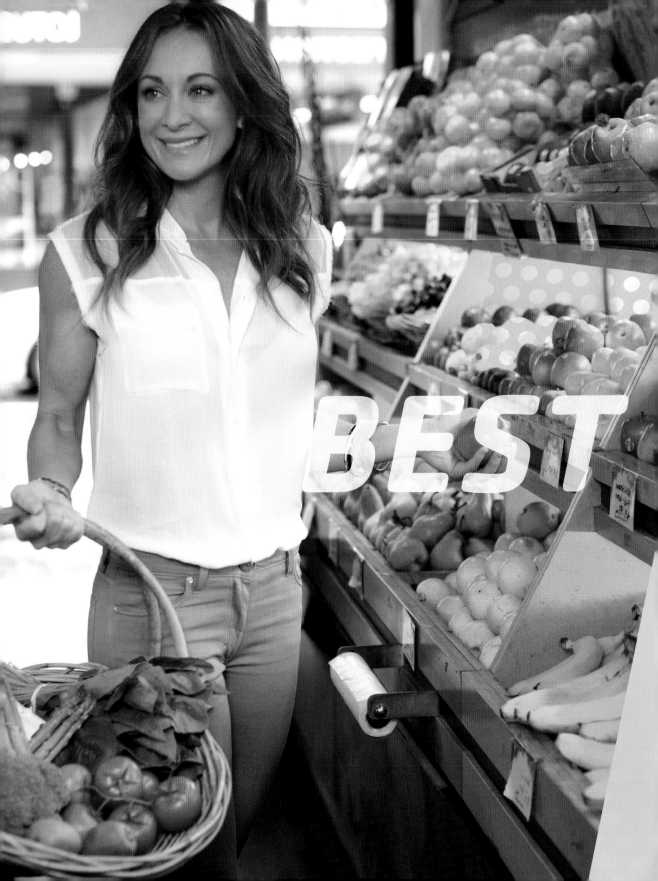

eating

Food is the fuel that drives you towards the best version of yourself that you can be. Making the right choices, getting all the essential nutrients your body requires and, of course, creating delicious meals are fundamental to a better, healthier lifestyle. Include my superfoods in your daily meal plan to get the best that nature can offer to improve and maintain your health. And they're all in my heavenly recipes.

GETTING YOUR DIET RIGHT

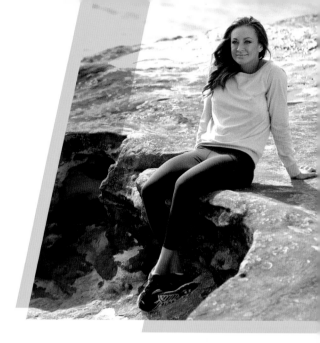

Even though exercise is a major part of my life, I know that when it comes to our health, what we put in our mouths is largely responsible for having a body that works well. Don't get me wrong – regular, well-programed training is linked to so many physical and emotional benefits, and I will always make it a part of my life. But to get the best out of ourselves, we need to be **putting the right fuel in the tank**.

Nourishing ourselves is a basic human task. We need to do it every few hours, and **the choices that we make can be the difference between good and poor health**.

Parents instinctively want the very best for their children, and teaching children how and what to eat is surely one of the most fundamental tasks that a parent can take on.

How then, as a society, have we allowed this most basic human activity to get so out of control? How can it be that so many of us are eating the wrong foods? And way too much of them? Why are we eating foods that, instead of supporting our physical selves, are actually detrimental to our health?

What we have allowed to happen is that we've left the responsibility of feeding ourselves to others. Food manufacturers, fast-food chains – their interest in our nutrition is secondary to the profits that they make by selling us their products. And there's nothing wrong with that. Their role as a company, as a commercial operation, isn't to make the most nutritious food possible. It's to make profits, because if they didn't make any money they wouldn't exist.

But our role as human beings trying to be the best physical version of ourselves is to nourish ourselves, and our children, with the most nutritious food available. To do that, we can't afford to give control of what we eat to others. **We must take back the power and responsibility for what we eat.**

So, I want to give you information and recipes that mean you can make the best, positive choices for fuelling this amazing creation – your body.

And, of course, the recipes put together for this book are not just nutritious – they're delicious!

With all of these recipes I have worked backwards. I started with the vitamins, minerals and nutrients that are most significant in supporting a healthy, exercising body and researched which foods were most packed with them. With this knowledge in the bag, the next step was to create gorgeous, tempting dishes from these wholefoods, dishes as delectable to eat as they are good for your body.

All of my recipes are, of course, carefully calorie-counted. They're also carefully worked out size-wise. **Portion size is just as critical** as which foods you put on your plate – getting used to eating a sensible amount of food at each sitting is important for optimal health, as well as for keeping your weight firmly under control.

Physical activity, rigorous exercise, and particularly strength training, is demanding on our bodies. All of our complex physiological processes are crying out for the nutrients they need to build, repair and restore. Think about it – how often have you seen people get sick with a cold or the flu two weeks or so into a new exercise regime? More often than not it's because their bodies have been so busy using vital nutrients to repair themselves that their immune systems have been compromised, and bang! Hello, sickbed!

> *The foods we eat affect every physiological process in the body. We owe it to ourselves to give our bodies the best, most nutritious fuel.*

These recipes include foods that are rich in iron, vitamin E and vitamin B12. Foods that are jam-packed with amino acids and essential fatty acids. And foods that are brimming with antioxidants and minerals. These are the **nutrients that we rely upon most** when we embark on a training program that pushes our muscles and organs to new levels. So it makes sense to get what we need of these indispensable nutrients from the foods most full of them.

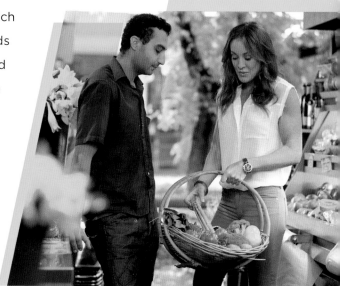

SUPERFOODS

The foods that I have selected for the recipes don't just have a smattering of these nutrients – they are crammed with them. They are the foods that have the highest representation of energy-producing, tissue-repairing, immune system-supporting nutrients that you can readily buy. They are the exerciser's true superfoods.

The expression 'superfood' gets used quite a lot these days, and even though most of the time I agree with the 'superfood' label, there are quite a few times that I don't.

For me, there are four criteria a food has to fulfil to be considered 'super'.

Firstly, **a true superfood must be readily available** at your local supermarket or greengrocer. If you've got to travel all over the place to find it, then the 'super' bit starts to lose its gloss.

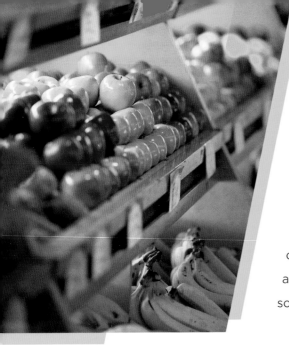

A superfood also has to be calorie-effective, meaning that it's **naturally low in calories** and you don't have to eat half a kilo of it to get the desired nutrient effect.

Next, it has to be **inexpensive**. Foods that are touted as 'superfoods' frequently could be called 'super-priced foods', and getting whacked at the checkout usually means that you'll never buy it again. A real superfood is one that you eat routinely, so that rules out expensive hard-to-get items.

Lastly, the information about a superfood's nutritional qualities must be **more than marketing hype**. There are lots of so-called 'miracle' food stories but, frankly, I don't believe that lifetime wolfberry enthusiast Li Ching-Yuen lived to the ripe old age of 252 years, and I suggest that you don't either.

So, my superfood list comprises the foods that fit not one or two, but *all* these criteria.

There are a lot of 'top ten superfoods' lists published, but it's important to remember that there are lots of different testing methods, so there will always be a variation in the results. For my money, a superfood needs to deliver upward of 50 per cent of the recommended daily allowance of two or three important nutrients to get on the list in the first place.

Now this doesn't mean that all the other amazing wholefoods that aren't on this list shouldn't be on your menu. On the contrary, they should be eaten and enjoyed daily. It's just that the foods listed below deliver **extraordinary quantities of nutrients**. They are truly superfoods.

Surround yourself with the superfoods on my list. Incorporating them into your diet everyday will ensure your body is getting fabulous nutritional value with few calories.

THE MICHELLE BRIDGES SUPERFOODS

VEGETABLES

ASPARAGUS / Asparagus is a great antioxidant and anti-inflammatory. Best of all, though, it's really versatile, so you can eat it raw, grilled, steamed, whatever. It spoils quickly so stand the spears in an inch of water and keep in the fridge until just before cooking.

SPINACH / Could spinach be the world's healthiest vegetable? Like asparagus it's rich in antioxidants and packed with flavonoids, making it a big hitter in the anti-inflammatory department. It's an anti-cancer superstar.

SILVERBEET / Another green leafy vegetable champion, chocker with vitamins A, C and K, and runner-up to spinach as the world's healthiest vegetable. Store it in the fridge in those opaque plastic bags that some cereals come in to keep it crisp and yummy.

MUSHROOMS / I love how mushies can be eaten with everything, cooked or raw, in salads or vegetable bakes. They are a wicked antioxidant, and anti-inflammatory too. Mushrooms are rich in the anti-cancer chemical selenium. Store in the fridge, as they will spoil quickly.

BROCCOLI / A great detoxifier and packed with vitamins C and K, along with a long list of other nutrients, and another anti-cancer hero. It'll also help to get your cholesterol in check - steaming is the best cooking method to retain as many of these properties as possible.

BRUSSELS SPROUTS / Vitamins A, C and K top a long list of nutrients present in brussels sprouts. Steaming is the best preparation, but don't overcook them – when they're soft and mushy they've lost both flavour and nutrients. Store in the bottom drawer of the fridge.

FISH

SARDINES / High on my list of convenience foods come sardines. These are a great sustainable source of protein, heart-healthy omega-3s and bone-supporting vitamin D. If you get them fresh, cook straightaway. I like them rolled in flour and grilled or pan-fried with a little olive oil. A squeeze of lemon, a splash of balsamic, and bingo!

SALMON / Readily available and delicious, salmon is also an omega-3 and protein heavyweight. Antioxidant, anti-inflammatory and immune-system supportive, the list goes on for this true superfood.

SUPERFOODS

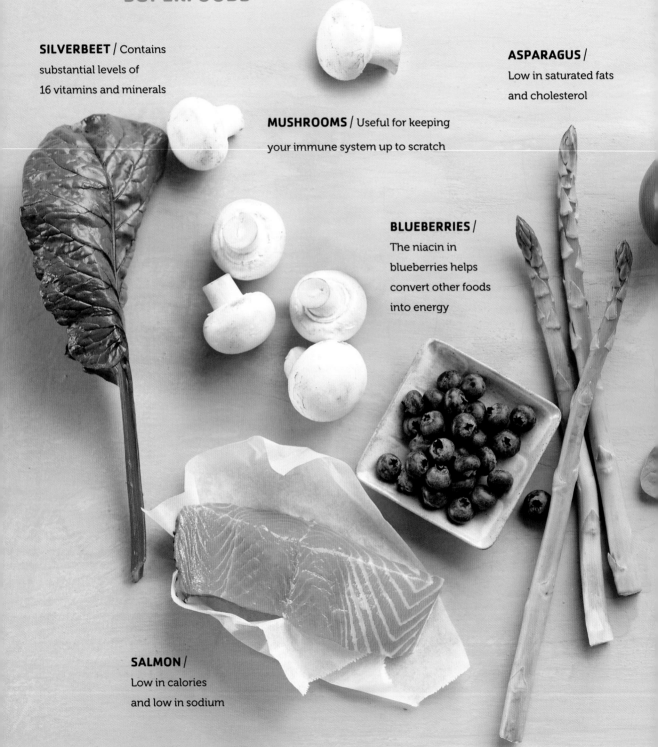

SILVERBEET / Contains substantial levels of 16 vitamins and minerals

MUSHROOMS / Useful for keeping your immune system up to scratch

ASPARAGUS / Low in saturated fats and cholesterol

BLUEBERRIES / The niacin in blueberries helps convert other foods into energy

SALMON / Low in calories and low in sodium

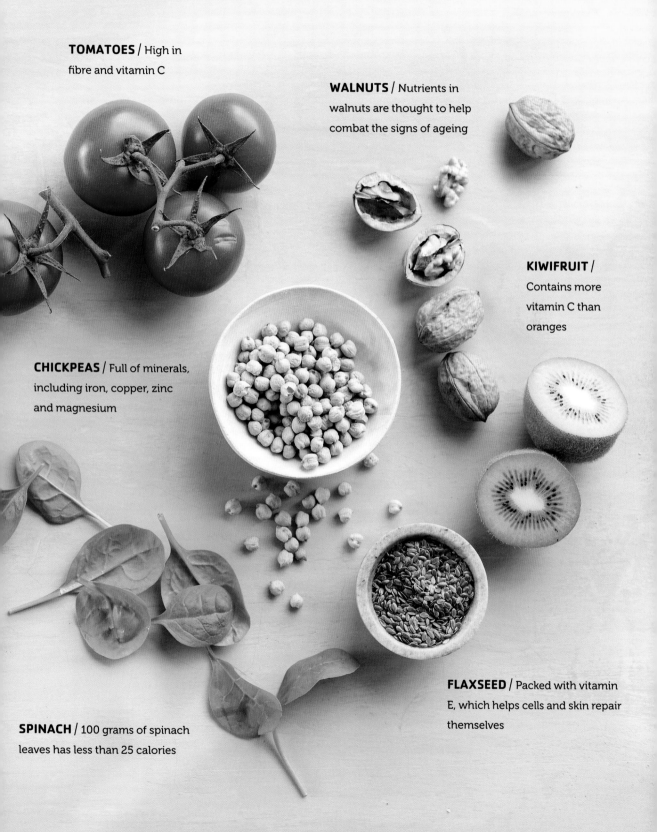

TOMATOES / High in fibre and vitamin C

WALNUTS / Nutrients in walnuts are thought to help combat the signs of ageing

KIWIFRUIT / Contains more vitamin C than oranges

CHICKPEAS / Full of minerals, including iron, copper, zinc and magnesium

FLAXSEED / Packed with vitamin E, which helps cells and skin repair themselves

SPINACH / 100 grams of spinach leaves has less than 25 calories

FRUIT

KIWIFRUIT / Kiwifruit is almost a vitamin C pill, there's so much of it in each one. As well as being a great antioxidant, kiwifruit has a particular ability to support our DNA. Wait until they ripen fully before eating.

ORANGES / Apart from looking fabulous in a fruit bowl, oranges are well known for their vitamin C content. Don't worry about picking out the white pith between the segments too much as it too is packed with nutrients.

BLUEBERRIES / I love a handful of bloobs. Whereas some antioxidants tend to be more supportive of particular organs or body systems, blueberries support all of the body systems, making them the number one fruit superfood in my book. They are versatile too – add them to breakfast cereal, salads and yoghurt.

TOMATOES / Thankfully we're no longer burdened with those bloated watery things we used to get years ago; these days there are a variety of these rich sources of antioxidants and nutrients available. Cooked or raw, they are always in my kitchen for their anti-cancer properties (particularly prostate and breast cancer).

NUTS, GRAINS & SEEDS

WHEATGERM / Wheatgerm is the part of the wheat that is discarded along with the husk during processing. A bit silly really, since it's the part with the most nutritional value. I love it because it's a concentrated dose of nutrients that I can use in muesli or scatter on a salad. You can even add it to a protein drink.

OATS / Oats have a unique cardiovascular-health-protecting property, and for my money they are the best breakfast cereal around. Unlike wheat, most of the nutrients remain in the grain when they are hulled, so use them for porridge or homemade muesli, or to beef up a protein shake.

WALNUTS / These cholesterol-decreasing nuts are brimming with omega-3 fatty acids. They are always available and taste great in salads or crushed over breakfast cereal, or even as a filling snack. They are quite high in calories, but don't be put off by that – in small servings their anti-inflammatory properties have been shown to support weight loss.

FLAXSEED / Big on antioxidants and brimming with omega-3, flaxseed is a wicked food source for supporting your cardiovascular system. They're not always easy to include in your daily diet though, so be creative – sprinkle on breakfast cereal, fruit platters or yoghurt, and use when you're baking.

BEANS AND LENTILS

CHICKPEAS / Like flaxseed, chickpeas keep well. They are fantastic for digestion and for regulating blood-sugar levels, as well as being very rich in folate and fibre. Use them in soups and salads.

MEAT

KANGAROO / I've been eating kangaroo for years now, and I'm a big believer in its high-protein, low-fat and high-iron properties. Kangaroo is also a great low-calorie meat, with around the same calories per gram as white fish.

CALVES' LIVER / This might seem like an odd superfood, but it would never have made it to this list if it weren't an absolute cracker. Calves' liver is full of protein, has stratospheric levels of vitamins A, B12 and copper, and supports your immune system, your cardiovascular system and colonic health. A true superfood. If you haven't tried it, do.

EGGS / Eggs got a bad rap a few years ago because they are high in cholesterol, but it has since been shown that we can eat one or two eggs a day and actually improve our cholesterol profile. Eggs are a fantastic source of protein as well as brain-supporting selenium and a load of other micronutrients. They are always available and can be used in all kinds of cooking – a definite superfood.

DAIRY

YOGHURT / Yoghurt boosts the immune system, lowers cholesterol and helps with weight management. It's a super snack that is a worthy inclusion on my superfoods list. There are loads of yoghurts available (look for one with high levels of acidophilus, bifidobacterium and casei bacteria), and when cooking you can use it instead of cream in some dishes. It's also a great topping for fruit dishes, and as a base for salad dressings.

SUPERFOODS

SARDINES / One sardine contains only about 25 calories

YOGHURT / A good way to get protein and calcium into your diet

CALVES' LIVER / Has high levels of iron and selenium, a mineral that helps regulate the thyroid

KANGAROO / Contains less than two per cent fat and has high levels of zinc

BROCCOLI / This cruciferous vegetable has anti-cancer properties

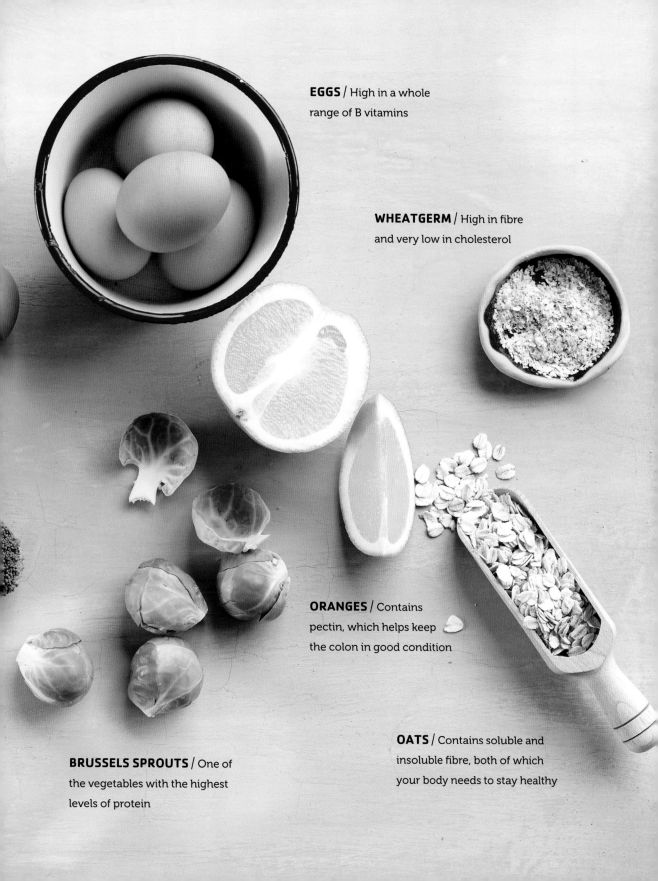

EGGS / High in a whole range of B vitamins

WHEATGERM / High in fibre and very low in cholesterol

ORANGES / Contains pectin, which helps keep the colon in good condition

OATS / Contains soluble and insoluble fibre, both of which your body needs to stay healthy

BRUSSELS SPROUTS / One of the vegetables with the highest levels of protein

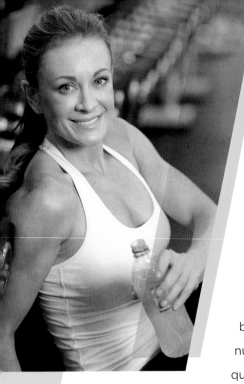

CHOICES /

What we eat is largely a product of our environment – our social and personal environments.

If you take a long hard look at our social environment – service stations that serve as shopfronts for fast-food chains, and Australian suburbs full of fast-food restaurants, many of them with drive-throughs – well, you don't need me to tell you that it's pretty tough out there.

There have never been so many cheap calories available, but most of the time these calories are not packed with nutrients, and often they are very unhealthy options. Let's be quite clear – we will never get on top of the obesity crisis that grips much of the Western world as long as the current fast-food situation remains as it is today. Changing our social environment is slow and costly, and usually takes proactive government initiatives like restricting junk-food advertising and limiting the number of outlets.

Changes to our personal environment, however, are much easier and can be undertaken a hell of a lot quicker. An easy first step – simply drag your wheelie bin into your kitchen, and start chucking!

When it comes down to it, **we all have a choice to make every time we eat**. It's not complicated – it simply means that when we have a meal or a snack, we should **make a conscious choice about what we will eat**. Or not eat. I call this 'intentional eating'. It means eating with intent. It's not grabbing a 'whatever' out of the fridge as you walk past, or picking up a nutty-honey-muesli-loggy thingy on a whim when you fill up at the servo.

It involves thinking about what you're going to eat, and when you're going to eat it, and then making whatever arrangements you need to make it happen. You need to make active, intentional choices about your food.

Critically, for intentional eating to take place, you need to be organised.

Here are a few tips to help:

- You need to **set some rules** in your house. For example, in our house (and *The Biggest Loser* house), no one is allowed to eat when they are either standing up or sitting on the couch. This stops unintentional eating – eating should only be done at the table.
- You need to **have an apple in your bag** when you walk out of the door in the morning. And a shopping list if you're dropping into the supermarket to pick up some groceries on the way home.
- You need to **avoid getting overly hungry**, so you don't inhale the entire breadbasket the moment the waiter puts it on the table in a restaurant.
- You need to **restrict your alcohol intake** to avoid that sinking feeling you get when you find the wrapper of a family block of chocolate on the couch next to an empty bottle of sauvignon blanc in the morning.

But don't just think of it as a lot of boring limitations – there's a joy in intentional eating. It's the joy of being in control, of holding the power over the basest of our daily tasks – feeding ourselves.

There are lots of companies that take online orders for home-delivered fresh food these days, which means that you can place a standing order of your most commonly used fruits and veggies and have them delivered to your door each week. That way you always have high-quality fresh food in your kitchen.

FEEDING YOUR BRAIN

Just as we can adjust our exercise regime to support brain health, we can eat to support it too. As a rule of thumb, any foods that are good for your heart are good for your brain as well. While changing your diet isn't going to see your IQ become stratospheric overnight, it will help to improve your memory and other cognitive functions. It can also reduce the risk of dementia.

A recent study by Dr. Felice Jacka from Victoria's Deakin University gives some fascinating insights into the **relationship between diet and cognitive function**. She interviewed more than 1000 women about their diet and mental health. Unlike other studies in the past, it wasn't just about the role of specific nutrients in mental health. It examined the subjects' whole diet as it related to depression and anxiety disorders.

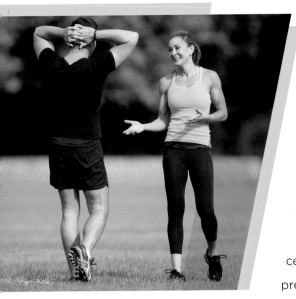

The study found that those subjects who had diets high in processed foods and junk food were more likely to suffer anxiety and depression disorders than those who – you guessed it – had wholefood diets high in vegetables, fruit, fish and lean protein. And the results were the same across all the subjects, irrespective of age and socio-economic status, or whether they were keen exercisers or more sedentary people.

Dr. Jacka also conducted a study on adolescents. Her results suggest that it may be possible to prevent teenage depression by adopting a nutritious, high-quality diet, with the potential knock-on effect of improved academic performance. Anything that can help our kids in these ways has got to be worth paying attention to, right?

Those kids whose diets got worse over the two years saw deterioration in their mental health – greater anxiety, more depression - as opposed to an improvement in mental health in those whose diet improved.

Even though the potential for positive improvement to mental health is enormous, we should remember that these adjustments are aimed at the most important organ in our bodies, our brains, so they shouldn't require a significant outcome to make them worthwhile. A modest improvement easily justifies **making conscious, and often delicious, changes to our diet**.

What we eat affects all the organs in the body, from the brain and heart to the skin and eyes. Eating nutritious wholefoods is good for the whole body.

BRAIN FOODS /

To give our brains a boost through what we eat, we need to consume foods that are full of certain key nutrients.

OMEGA-3 FATTY ACIDS

When Mum told you to eat your fish because it would make you brainy, she wasn't far off the mark. Omega-3 fatty acids, like those found in cold-water fish, help **fight against mental disorders** such as ADHD, dyslexia, dementia, depression, bipolar disorder and schizophrenia.

Omega-3s elevate the levels of a groovy little protein called brain-derived neurotrophic factor (BDNF to its friends). Harvard Psychiatrist Dr. John Ratey has described BDNF as 'the crucial biological link between thought, emotions and movement'. It stimulates brain-cell growth and also increases the signal strength between neurons, improving the cells' ability to talk to each other.

So BDNF is not something that you want to be running short of any time soon. And omega-3 cultivates more of it! How cool is that? Think of it as chook poo for the brain veggie patch. Taking an omega-3 supplement is good, but eating foods rich in omega-3 is even better because they usually come with a load of other nutrients as well.

The Michelle Bridges Omega-3 All Stars are:

- salmon
- mackerel
- sardines
- prawns
- kiwifruit
- flaxseed
- walnuts

Flaxseed and walnuts are great because you can add them to lots of different dishes. You can sprinkle them on pasta dishes, add them to salads or bake
them in muffins – the list is endless.

They are particularly great at breakfast time, added to your muesli. Slice
some kiwifruit on as well (kiwifruit seeds are rich in alpha-linolenic acid, an
omega-3 fatty acid) and you've got a slammin' brainy breakfast.

FOLATE

My next fave brain nutrient is folate. Folate is **crucial in the development of
new cells**, especially when you're going through periods of rapid cell division,
like infancy and pregnancy.

Folate deficiency is a marker of the neuropathology for Alzheimer's disease, which is medi-speak for 'EAT YOUR GREENS!' You also risk an increased
likelihood of depression or other neurological disorders if you are short of
folate, so get some into your diet every day. It's that important.

The Michelle Bridges Folate All Stars are:

- avocado
- asparagus
- beans
- beetroot
- broccoli
- cauliflower
- corn
- cos lettuce
- peas
- spinach
- lentils
- liver

MAGNESIUM

Magnesium is another brain-food fave. It is **involved in over 300 metabolic
functions of the body**, a large percentage of which are crucial to cognitive
function, activating key enzymes that allow your brain function. It's really, really
important. But many of us are deficient, mostly because of our Western diets
that don't often include magnesium-rich foods. And foods that are high in

sugar and salt can actually lower the level of magnesium in our bodies. Stress is also known to deplete magnesium stores.

But of all the things known to deplete magnesium, alcohol is by far the most efficient. It's magnesium deficiency that is responsible for the infamous (and sometimes life-threatening) 'DTs', and emergency rooms routinely stock injections of magnesium sulfate to treat alcohol overdoses.

Magnesium occurs in lots of foods but usually only in small amounts. So we need to eat a variety of these foods because, unlike trace elements like zinc, it's not easy to get your daily dose of magnesium from one food source.

The Michelle Bridges Magnesium All Stars are:

- wheat bran
- spinach
- silverbeet
- almonds
- soybeans
- cashew nuts
- peanuts
- oatmeal
- brown rice
- pinto beans
- baked potato (yes, even the humble spud is a good source of magnesium!)

ZINC

Zinc may be last on my list of favourite brain nutrients but don't let that fool you. Apart from playing a critical role in brain plasticity (the ability of the brain to develop over time), zinc is anti-bacterial, anti-viral, anti-cancer, anti-oxidation and anti-fungal. Like magnesium, it's involved in over 300 processes in the body, particularly in our reproductive and immune systems, and holds the title for having **the widest range of essential functions** of all the trace elements.

Many of us are zinc-deficient, as it gets lost when foods are refined. Alcohol, sugar, smoking and the contraceptive pill also increase our zinc loss, but it's crucial for healthy living and for getting our best bodies. It is to the human body what shoes are to the modern woman. Need I say more?

The Michelle Bridges Zinc All Stars are:

- oysters (gold star for oysters – one oyster will supply your entire recommended daily allowance of zinc!)
- prawns
- lobster
- ginger root
- lamb
- pecan nuts
- dry split peas
- green peas
- turnips
- Brazil nuts
- egg yolks
- rye
- oats
- peanuts
- almonds

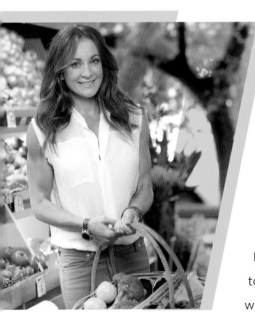

You'll notice in this book that all of the workouts feature free-form resistance exercises to activate the cerebellum, and that where possible all of the recipes feature foods rich in omega-3 essential fatty acids, folate, magnesium and zinc. I have designed them this way so that the most important organ in your body gets the attention it deserves. Happy brain boosting!

EATING FOR HEART HEALTH

Now, I'm no biochemist, nor am I a dietician. But I do like to have a basic understanding of the nutrients in food and what they can do for our bodies, and I recommend that you do as well. **Knowledge is one of the best ways of taking the power back** over our diet choices. For instance, when it comes to heart health, there are a few ingredients that are standouts for the nutritional benefits they give us.

A day with a good workout, lots of incidental activity and three nutritious meals is like a visit to the spa for your body and mind.

HEART FOODS /

OMEGA–3 FATTY ACIDS

You've already read about the role of omega-3 fatty acids on page 105 when it comes to brain health, but they are equally **crucial when it comes to your heart**. Because the human body can't make them itself, we need to make good food choices to ensure we get enough of this essential nutrient.

WHERE / Oily fish like sardines, tuna, salmon and mackerel, shellfish such as green-lipped mussels, oysters and crab (seafood has the additional benefit of being low in fat, further promoting heart health), flaxseed, eggs, grass-fed red meat, walnuts, and canola, soybean and walnut oils.

BEST EATEN / Oily fish two to three times a week, red meat once a week, one egg per day. Try to use oils that are high in omega-3s in place of olive oil or vegetable oil when appropriate to the dish.

WHY / Omega-3s are superstars when it comes to cardiovascular health. They stabilise heart rhythm and help to lower your heart rate. They also make your blood less sticky, reducing the risk of clots and blocked arteries and, in doing so, **reduce the risk of a heart attack or stroke**. They also help improve blood-vessel elasticity, another weapon in the fight against heart disease. By lowering the amount of fat-carrying triglycerides in your blood, omega-3s also lower the potential for artery-blocking plaque deposits. They increase the quantity of high-density lipoproteins (HDL) in your body, which help remove cholesterol from your blood. Busy little buggers, aren't they?

HERO STATUS / We're only just starting to realise the importance of omega-3 fatty acids to our health. By way of example, DHA (docosahexaenoic acid), one of the most important omega-3s, is not only essential to cardiovascular health, but is the primary structural component of the brain's cerebral cortex, retinas, sperm and testicles. It is also a crucial component in breastmilk, helping nursing babies develop eye and brain tissue.

CAROTENOIDS

Carotenoids are responsible for the colour of vegetables, which is why nutritionists are always banging on about having lots of different coloured veggies on your plate.

WHERE / Carrots, sweet potatoes, spinach, kale, capsicum, tomatoes, papaya.

BEST EATEN / Daily, raw or lightly steamed.

WHY / Carotenoids **protect your cells** from free radicals and prop up your immune system, both of which are really important for exercisers. They also provide vitamin A and support your reproductive system.

HERO STATUS / Carotenoids have been shown to improve cell communication (picture billions of cells texting – cute!) This helps prevent irregular cell growth, also known as cancer. Their antioxidants can help to slow the ageing process.

FLAVONOIDS

Flavonoids are pigments that, like carotenoids, give fruits and vegetables their colour. There are over 6000 different kinds and they're found in virtually all plant life.

WHERE / Apples, apricots, blueberries, pears, raspberries, strawberries, black beans, cabbage, onions, parsley, pinto beans, tomatoes.

BEST EATEN / Daily. Keep cooking to a minimum as overcooking leaches flavonoids from foods.

WHY / Flavonoids scour the body for the unused oxygen molecule that's left behind messing up other cells after oxygen is used as fuel. They are anti-inflammatory and elevate the potency of another major antioxidant, vitamin C. They may also play a role in cancer prevention.

HERO STATUS / They are **awesome antioxidants** that not only fight cell damage in their own right, but also combine with other nutrients to increase their effectiveness.

FIBRE

There are two types of fibre. Insoluble fibre is the one found in vegetable skins and whole wheat that makes your poo bulky and pass quickly through your system. But here I'm talking about soluble fibre, which attracts water during digestion. Like the insoluble kind, it's good for your colon, but also helps maintain a healthy heart.

WHERE / Oats, barley, nuts, fruit, blueberries, celery, peas, beans, legumes.

BEST EATEN / Start every day with oats, nuts and fruit for brekkie.

WHY / Soluble fibre can help **get your LDL blood cholesterol levels down**. This is the 'bad' cholesterol that deposits plaque on the artery walls and can mean your tissues don't get the blood and oxygen they need.

HERO STATUS / Soluble fibre is digested slowly meaning you feel fuller for longer. It can also help with insulin sensitivity, important for those of us who are watching our blood sugar levels. These two features make fibre a really important part of the weight-loss equation.

FOLATE

Folate is a B-group vitamin (B9, to be precise) and it's involved in the **production of new cells** and has a particularly important role in the repair and function of DNA. But it also has a vital role in maintaining cardiovascular health.

WHERE / Beef liver, avocados, beetroot, cauliflower, walnuts, hazelnuts, spinach, asparagus, beans, peas.

BEST EATEN / Daily.

WHY / Folate helps to reduce homocysteine levels in the blood. Homocysteine is an amino acid that, when its level gets elevated, can attack coronary artery walls making it easy for blood clots to form, which may lead to a heart attack.

HERO STATUS / Anything that is anti-cancer, anti-cardiovascular disease and keeps DNA in good shape has got my vote.

Do not skip brekkie! That's an order. A lot of people think that not eating in the a.m. is an easy way to get ahead in their weight loss. But it really is false economy. You need a good, healthy breakfast every morning to kick-start your metabolism, give you energy for the day ahead and to fill you up so that you don't feel tempted to pick up an unhealthy snack mid-morning. Here are a few of my favourite, tried-and-tested dishes for giving you the best start to the day.

Spiced pear and ricotta toast

This delicious brekkie takes just 5 minutes to prepare – that's less time than it takes to make a pot of tea. If it's a chilly morning, warm up the ricotta mix for a few seconds in the microwave – it will help to melt the honey.

SERVES 2 | *PREP* 5 mins | *CAL PER SERVE* 353

4 slices wholegrain bread

200 g low-cal ricotta

2 teaspoons honey

¼ teaspoon ground ginger

1 pear, cored and sliced

ground cinnamon

1 | Toast the bread.

2 | Meanwhile, combine the ricotta, honey and ginger in a bowl.

3 | Spread the ricotta mixture over the toast and top with pear slices. Sprinkle with cinnamon to serve.

TIP | Use a little freshly grated ginger instead of the ground kind for added zing.

Homemade muesli with yoghurt

You can prepare this at the weekend so it's ready for the week ahead. If you don't fancy making your own, grab a bag of untoasted muesli from the grocer that fits your calorie target (it should be no more that 350 calories per 100 grams). Beware the ones with buckets of dried fruit as they're super sweet and full of sulphur, though if the rest of it looks OK you could always pick out the fruit.

SERVES 4 / *PREP* 5 mins / *CAL PER SERVE* 300

2 cups rolled oats

½ cup bran

⅓ cup sunflower seeds

⅓ cup pumpkin seeds

100 g pitted dates, chopped

¼ dried currants

1 cup skimmed milk or
   low-cal yoghurt, to serve

1 / Combine all the ingredients except the milk or yoghurt and store in an airtight container.

2 / Place half a cup of muesli in a bowl and add the skimmed milk or yoghurt or both to serve.

VARIATION / Serve with strawberries or grapes – they're low in calories and delicious.

Egg-white omelette with garlic mushrooms

Nothing beats this high-protein, low-calorie breakfast that combines two of my superfoods. You can leave one egg yolk in the mix, but that will add 50–70 calories (depending on the size of the egg) to your daily count.

SERVES 2 / *PREP* 10 mins / *COOK* 10 mins / *CAL PER SERVE* 300

olive oil spray

250 g mixed fresh mushrooms
   (oyster, Swiss brown, shimeji), sliced

1 garlic clove, crushed

2 tablespoons freshly chopped parsley

1 shallot, finely chopped

10 egg whites

freshly ground black pepper

4 slices wholegrain bread

1 | Lightly spray a frying pan with oil and heat on medium–high. Cook the mushrooms for 6 minutes, stirring, until browned. Stir in the garlic, parsley and shallot and cook for 30 seconds until fragrant. Remove from the heat.

2 | Whisk the egg whites in a bowl until combined. Stir through the mushroom mixture and season to taste with pepper.

3 | Toast the bread. Meanwhile, lightly spray a medium non-stick frying pan with olive oil and heat on medium–high. Pour in half of the egg-white mixture and cook for 1–2 minutes until just set. Fold over and slide onto a warm plate. Keep warm. Repeat with the remaining egg-white mixture for the second omelette.

4 | Serve the omelettes with the toast alongside.

Apple and pear porridge with cinnamon

The apple and pear add a delicious twist to this porridge. Great after a morning workout in winter!

SERVES 2 | *PREP* 10 mins | *COOK* 10 mins | *CAL PER SERVE* 332

1 cup rolled oats

2 tablespoons sultanas

1 large pear, cored

1 large green apple, coarsely grated

pinch of ground cinnamon

1 | Place the oats, sultanas and 2 cups of water into a small saucepan and bring it to the boil, then reduce the heat to low and cook the porridge for 5 minutes, stirring occasionally.

2 | Meanwhile, dice half of the pear and slice the rest.

3 | Stir the grated apple and diced pear into the porridge. Divide between two bowls, top with the sliced pear and sprinkle with cinnamon.

TIP | You don't need to peel the apple or pear in this recipe – the skins add some extra crunch and fibre.

Sesame chicken and spinach rice-paper rolls

I love making these at the table when guests come over for a relaxed weekend lunch. It's kinda fun that everyone digs in and makes their own; and kids love getting involved! It can get a little messy, but that's part of the fun. Oh, and they just happen to taste *great*!

SERVES 2 (6 rolls) / *PREP* 30 mins / *COOK* 5 mins / *CAL PER SERVE* 396

2 tablespoons sesame seeds

150 g cooked chicken, shredded

¼ × 250 g packet rice vermicelli noodles

100 g snow peas, thinly sliced

½ cup bean sprouts, tails removed

¼ red onion, thinly sliced

40 g baby spinach, shredded

½ cup mint, coarsely chopped

6 round rice paper sheets
 (22 cm in diameter)

1 / Put a saucepan of water on to boil. Meanwhile, heat a large frying pan on medium, add the sesame seeds and cook for 1–2 minutes until golden. Remove the pan from the heat and add the chicken, tossing and pressing down to coat well with the seeds. Set aside to cool.

2 / Add the noodles to the boiling water and cook for 2 minutes until tender. Drain, rinse under cold water and drain again. Combine the noodles, cooled chicken, snow peas, bean sprouts, onion, spinach and mint in a bowl.

3 / Fill a large bowl or roasting pan with room-temperature water, and soak the rice paper sheets for 30 seconds each, one at a time, until soft. Lift out each sheet and place on a clean tea towel to absorb any excess moisture.

4 / Spoon a sixth of the vermicelli mixture onto the lower half of one softened rice paper sheet. Fold the paper over the filling at the top and bottom, then fold the left and right sides over the filling and roll it up tightly. Cover the finished roll with a damp tea towel, to prevent it from drying out. Repeat with the remaining rice paper sheets and filling.

TIPS / This recipe is a great way to use up any leftover cooked chicken, but if you don't have any, you can also quickly char-grill or pan-fry a chicken breast. / Keep an eye on the rice paper sheets when you're soaking them: left in the water too long, they get too soft and will tear easily.

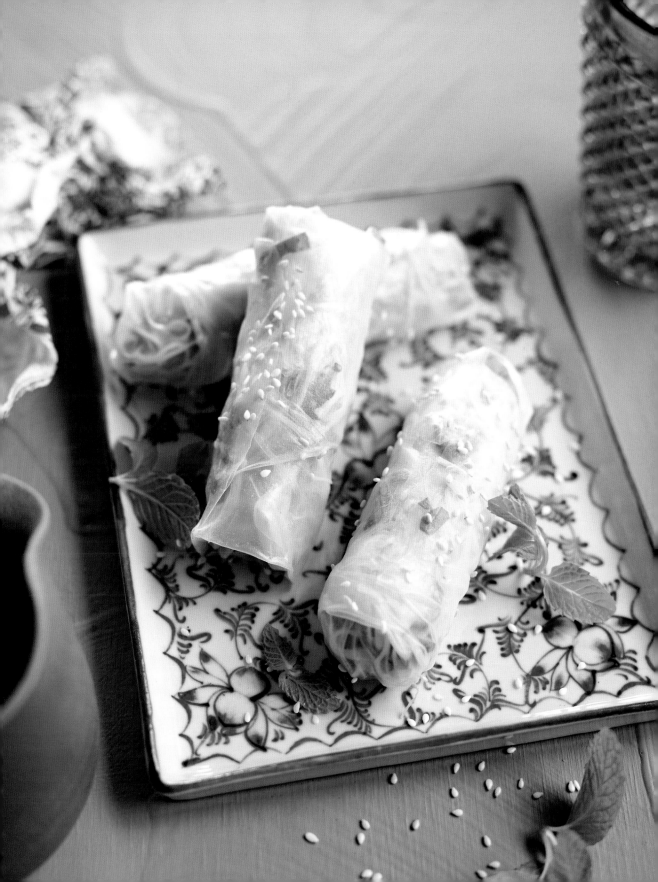

Egg, chive and fetta wrap

This is my new and improved take on what was my favourite sandwich as a child, the old egg and lettuce! Filling, tasty, easy to prepare and full of nutrients – yep, it ticks all my boxes!

SERVES 2 (2 wraps) | *PREP* 15 mins | *COOK* 10 mins | *CAL PER SERVE* 370

3 large eggs
100 g low-cal fetta cheese, crumbled
100 g low-cal cottage cheese
1 bunch chives, finely chopped

cracked black pepper
2 slices mountain bread
60 g watercress
1 Lebanese cucumber, cut into ribbons

1 | In a small saucepan of boiling water, cook the eggs for 6 minutes, then place into cold water. When they're cool enough to handle, peel the eggs and place into a medium bowl. Coarsely mash with the back of a fork. Stir in the fetta, cottage cheese and chives, and season with pepper.

2 | Spread the egg mixture over the mountain bread, then top with the watercress and cucumber. Roll the bread up tightly to enclose the filling. Halve each roll with a sharp knife before serving.

TIP | Watercress wilts very quickly, so use it the same day you buy it and make a small salad out of any leftover leaves.

VARIATIONS | Try adding 100 g of thinly sliced red capsicum for some crunch (384 calories per serve). | You can use herbs such as mint, parsley or basil instead of the chives if you prefer. | If you can't find any watercress, use rocket instead for a similarly peppery taste.

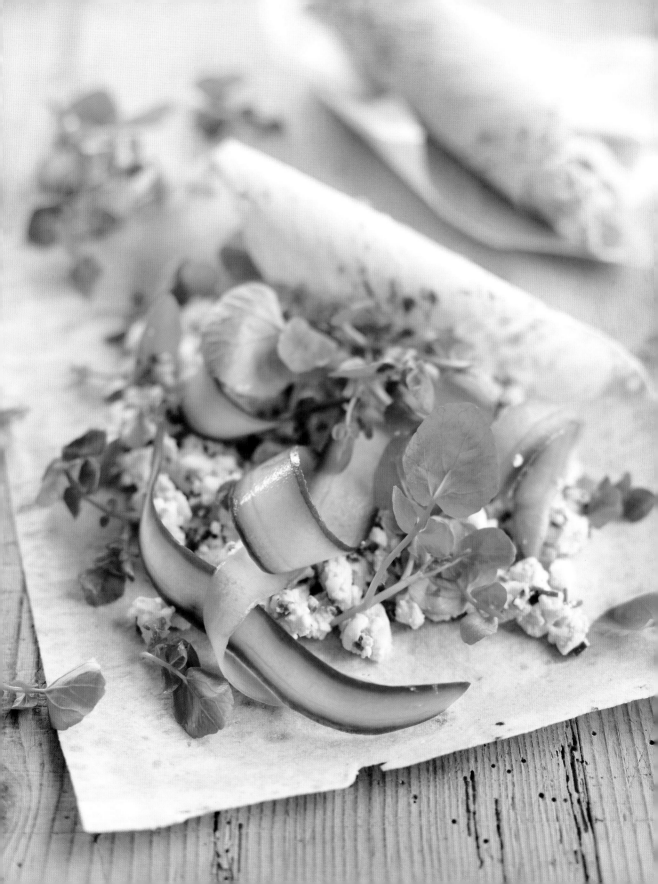

Sardine salad sandwich

Let me just put it out there: I LOVE sardines! Yes, they can be an acquired taste, but how good are these little suckers for you?! Jam-packed with both nutrients and omega-3s, they're brain and heart food. I'm bursting with energy just thinking about eating this!

SERVES 2 | *PREP* 15 mins | *CAL PER SERVE* 392

120 g canned sardines in olive oil, drained

1/3 cup cannellini beans, drained and rinsed

1 tablespoon lemon juice

2 tablespoons finely chopped parsley

1 spring onion, finely chopped

cracked black pepper

4 slices wholemeal or seeded bread

1 tomato, sliced

1/2 Lebanese cucumber, sliced

100 g radish, thinly sliced

1 | Combine the sardines, beans and lemon juice in a blender and process until smooth, then stir in a tablespoon of water to loosen the texture. Add the parsley and spring onion, stir, and season with pepper.

2 | Toast or grill the bread. Spread all the slices with the sardine mixture, then layer the remaining ingredients over 2 slices of the bread and top with the other 2 slices, sardine-spread side down. Cut each sandwich on the diagonal before serving.

TIP | The sardine spread is also terrific as a dip: try serving it with a Lebanese cucumber, a red capsicum and a large stalk of celery all cut into batons, plus 8 grissini (358 calories per serve).

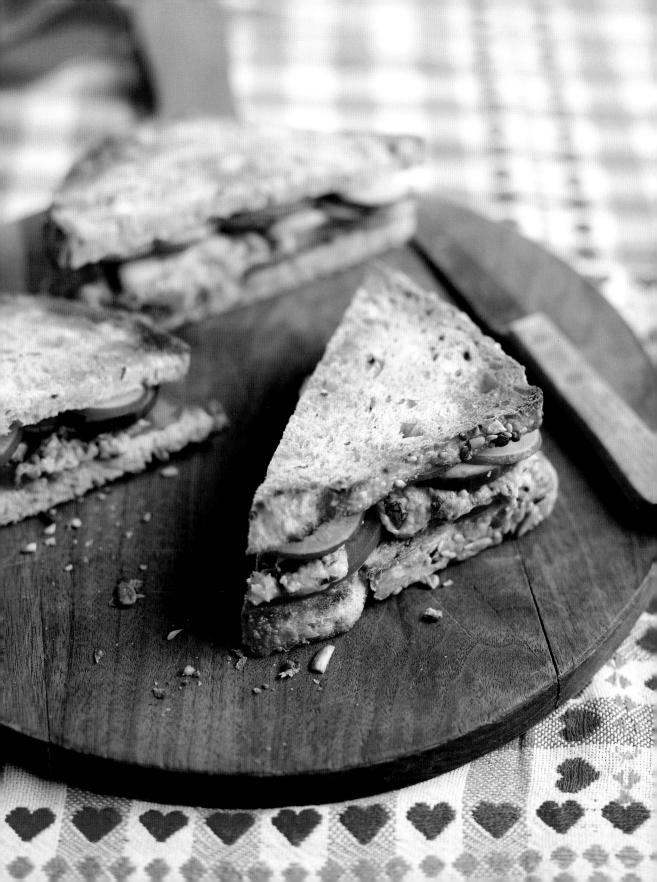

Tomato, mushroom and parsley bruschetta

Okay, I'm back in Italy with this one. It's a fabulous lunch that can be easily scaled up to serve a whole troop. Visually I find this a really special little dish; it looks like you've put in more effort than you actually have. Very yummy and I always feel good after I've eaten it.

SERVES 2 | *PREP* 10 mins | *COOK* 10 mins | *CAL PER SERVE* 358

3 teaspoons olive oil
2 cloves garlic, thinly sliced
1 bunch English spinach,
    washed and trimmed
200 g mushrooms, quartered

2 tomatoes, diced
2 tablespoons roughly chopped parsley
6 medium slices sourdough bread
cracked black pepper

1 | Heat 1 teaspoon of the oil in a large frying pan on medium–high. Cook the garlic for 30 seconds until it's fragrant and starts to colour. Add the spinach and cook, stirring, for 1 minute until wilted.

2 | Heat the remaining oil in the same pan on high. Cook the mushrooms for 4 minutes until browned and tender. Remove from the heat and mix with the tomatoes and parsley.

3 | Toast or grill the bread. Top each slice with the garlic spinach and then with the mushroom mixture. Season with pepper.

TIPS | Spinach often has a lot of grit, so make sure you wash it well. | Toss the mushrooms through the tomatoes and parsley just before you serve the bruschetta, so they don't start to cook and break down.

VARIATION | You can use this mushroom topping as the sauce for a quick pasta dish if you prefer. Cook 200 g of short pasta, drain, then stir through the hot mushroom mixture and sprinkle with 2 tablespoons of grated parmesan cheese (405 calories per serve).

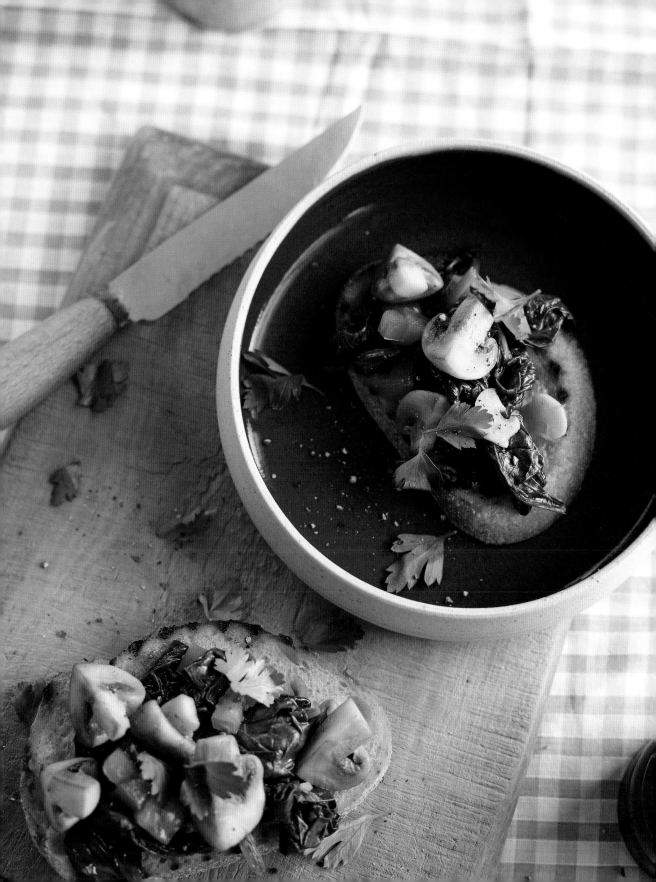

Grilled field mushrooms with thyme and fetta

Mushrooms are so meaty you really feel like you are getting good bang for your buck, even though they are low in calories. This is a great vegetarian dish with one of my favourite *super*foods in the starring role.

SERVES 2 | *PREP* 10 mins | *COOK* 10 mins | *CAL PER SERVE* 359

100 g low-cal fetta cheese
100 g low-cal ricotta cheese
1 clove garlic, crushed
2 teaspoons finely chopped fresh thyme
cracked black pepper
4 large flat field mushrooms

50 g sourdough bread, processed into
    breadcrumbs
50 g rocket
150 g cherry tomatoes, halved or quartered
2 teaspoons extra virgin olive oil
1 teaspoon balsamic vinegar

1 | Preheat the grill to high. Combine the fetta, ricotta, garlic and thyme in a small bowl. Season with pepper.

2 | Line an oven tray with foil, place the mushrooms on the tray, rounded-side up, and grill them, about 15 cm away from the heating element, for 5 minutes or until browned.

3 | Flip the mushrooms over, top with the cheese mixture and sprinkle with the breadcrumbs. Grill for a further 2–3 minutes until the breadcrumbs are golden and crisp.

4 | Meanwhile, combine the rocket and tomatoes in a large bowl. Drizzle with the oil and vinegar, season with pepper, then toss to coat.

5 | Serve the grilled mushrooms with the salad alongside.

TIPS | Breadcrumbs are handy for cooking, but you usually only need a slice or two's worth. If you've bought a loaf of your favourite bread and you know you'll be tempted to eat the leftovers, you can process the whole loaf into crumbs and store the unused crumbs in zip-lock bags in the freezer for next time. | Bread will crumble better if it's a day old, so slice it and leave overnight, covered with a tea towel, before processing.

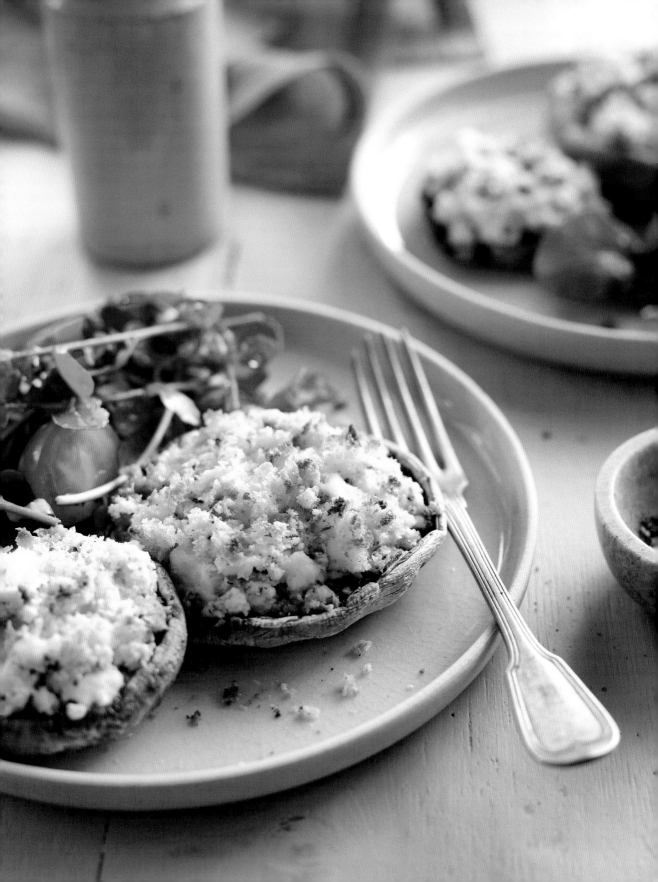

Cauliflower and quinoa salad

What a great combo of nutrients and protein this dish provides, while still being vegetarian. Yep, that's right, protein. Quinoa has the highest level of protein of any grain. It is also low-GI, and mixed into this salad it's a knockout.

SERVES 2 / *PREP* 15 mins / *COOK* 15 mins / *CAL PER SERVE* 357

⅓ cup quinoa, rinsed and drained
300 g cauliflower, coarsely grated
250 g cherry tomatoes, halved
150 g red capsicum, diced
1 small red onion, finely chopped
½ cup finely chopped mint

⅓ cup hazelnuts, toasted,
  coarsely chopped
1 tablespoon lemon juice
1 tablespoon olive oil
cracked black pepper

1 / Place the quinoa in a small saucepan with ⅔ cup of water. Bring to the boil, then reduce the heat and simmer, covered, for about 14 minutes or until the water is absorbed and the quinoa is tender. Allow to cool.

2 / Combine the quinoa with the remaining ingredients in a large bowl. Season with pepper and toss well, then serve.

TIPS / It's always a good idea to rinse quinoa thoroughly before cooking, as it can have a bitter taste. / This dish keeps well for 2–3 days in an airtight container in the fridge.

VARIATION / This salad is also lovely with grilled chicken breast (a quarter of the salad plus 150 g of chicken is 382 calories).

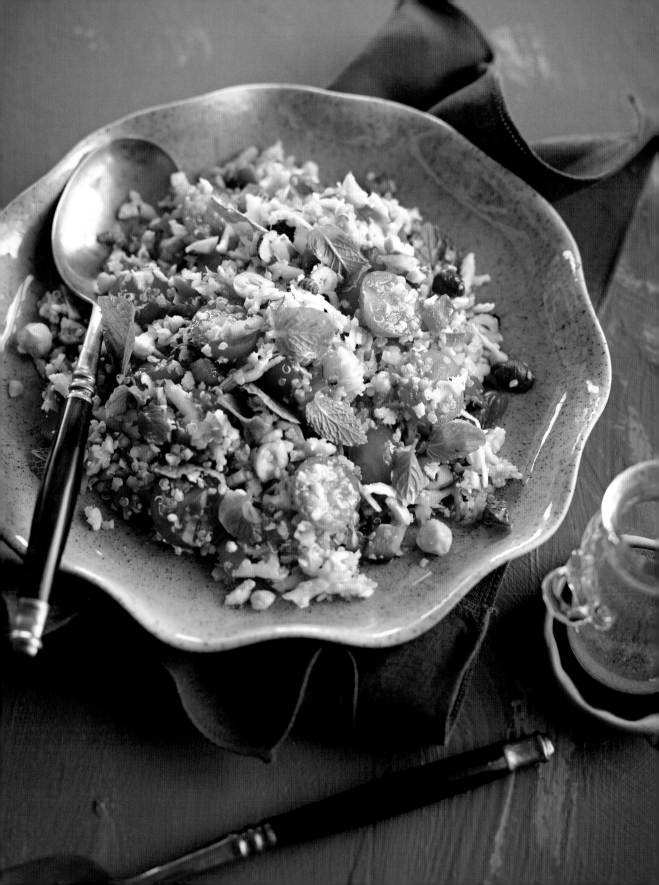

Grilled chicken and herbalicious salad with dried cranberries

Salad with crunchy chickpeas and dried cranberries: Yum! I experiment with my chickpeas for this one. Here I've oven-roasted them with a light drizzle of oil, but I have also used dried chickpeas soaked overnight, which makes them really nutty.

SERVES 2 / *PREP* 15 mins / *COOK* 25 mins / *CAL PER SERVE* 395

200 g canned chickpeas,
   drained and rinsed
½ teaspoon olive oil
olive oil spray
300 g skinless chicken breast fillet, trimmed
cracked black pepper
1 bunch asparagus, trimmed

50 g mesclun
1 cup parsley leaves
1 cup basil leaves, torn
½ cup mint leaves, torn
2 tablespoons dried cranberries
2 teaspoons extra virgin olive oil

1 / Preheat the oven to 220°C/200°C fan-forced.

2 / Pat the chickpeas dry with paper towel and discard the skins. Place the chickpeas in a small metal roasting pan and drizzle with the olive oil. Toss to coat well, then roast for 25 minutes, shaking the pan every 5 minutes, until golden and crunchy. Allow to cool in the pan.

3 / Meanwhile, lightly spray a char-grill pan with oil and heat on medium–high. Season the chicken with pepper, then cook on the grill for 8 minutes, turning halfway through, until lightly charred and cooked through. After 4 minutes, add the asparagus and cook for 4 minutes, turning, until lightly charred and tender.

4 / Remove the chicken and asparagus from the grill. Slice the chicken thinly and cut the asparagus into chunks. Combine the chicken, asparagus, mesclun, herbs, cranberries and chickpeas in a large bowl. Season with pepper, then drizzle with extra virgin olive oil and toss to coat before serving.

TIPS / Roast chickpeas make a delicious, crunchy, healthy snack, so why not roast the whole can and store the other half, after they've cooled, in an airtight container for later (148 calories)? / If your chicken breasts are particularly plump you may need to cook them for slightly longer.

128

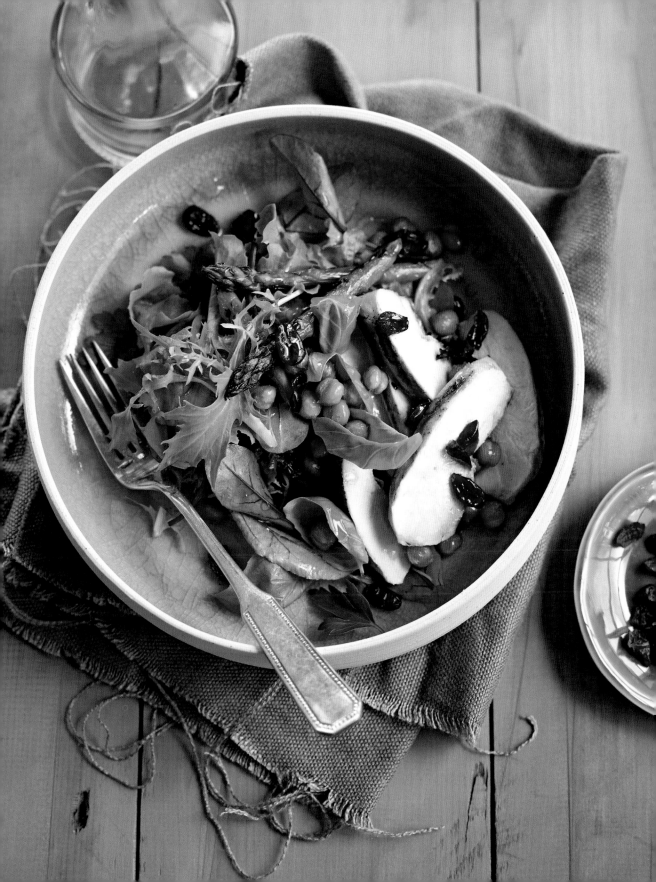

Slow-cooked beef stew with celeriac mash

This is a cracker for the weekend – the slow-cooking fills the kitchen with wonderful aromas. It's a low-fat meal that's rich in iron, zinc and vitamins, and is great for freezing.

SERVES 6 | *PREP* 20 mins | *COOK* 2 hrs 20 mins | *CAL PER SERVE* 390

1 tablespoon olive oil
300 g brown mushrooms, halved or
   quartered depending on size
1.2 kg gravy or chuck beef,
   trimmed and cut into 4 cm cubes
cracked black pepper
1 onion, chopped
3 cloves garlic, crushed
4 sprigs fresh thyme

1¼ cups low-salt beef stock
1 cup red wine
2 tablespoons low-salt tomato paste
1½ cups frozen peas
1.2 kg celeriac, peeled and
   cut into 4 cm cubes
½ cup low-cal ricotta cheese
chopped chives, to serve

1 | Preheat the oven to 200°C/180°C fan-forced.

2 | Heat half the oil in a heavy-based casserole dish on high, and cook the mushrooms for 5 minutes until browned. Set aside. Heat the remaining oil in the dish, then season the beef with pepper and cook it, in three batches, for 5 minutes per batch until well browned. Set the beef aside as well.

3 | Reduce the heat to medium. Add the onion, garlic and thyme and cook for 5 minutes, stirring, until softened. Add the stock, wine and tomato paste. Stir, scraping up any brown bits on the bottom of the pan, until the tomato paste has dissolved. Return the beef to the pan and bring the stew to the boil, then cover the dish, place it in the oven and cook for 1½ hours.

4 | Add the mushrooms, cover, and cook for another 20 minutes. Then stir in the peas and cook, covered, for 5 minutes. Discard the thyme sprigs.

5 | Meanwhile, over a saucepan of boiling water, steam the celeriac for 20 minutes, or until tender. Transfer to a large bowl, add the ricotta, and purée the mixture until smooth using a stick blender. Season with pepper.

6 | Divide the beef stew between six 1½-cup ramekins, top with mash and sprinkle with chives to serve.

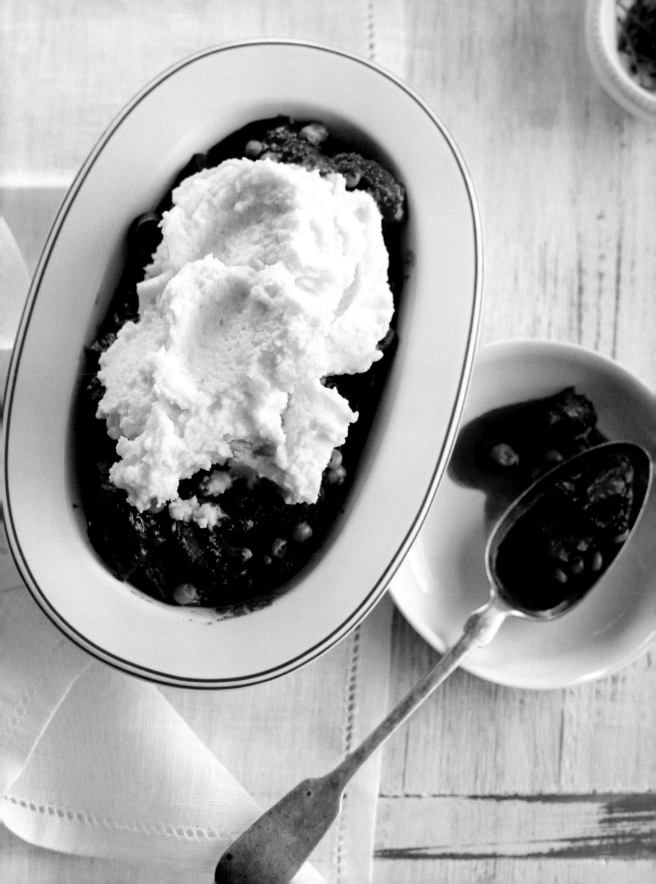

Kangaroo, orange and hazelnut salad

Fruit in salads is so my thing. A little sweet hit mixed with the crunch of nuts: I'm in heaven. Kangaroo – low in fat and cholesterol – is without doubt a superfood, and this is a really great way to introduce it into your diet.

SERVES 2 / *PREP* 15 mins / *COOK* 5 mins / *CAL PER SERVE* 376

2 oranges, segmented, juice reserved

2 teaspoons extra virgin olive oil

olive oil spray

250 g kangaroo fillet, trimmed

cracked black pepper

250 g witlof, leaves separated

50 g baby rocket

2 tablespoons mint leaves, torn

⅓ cup hazelnuts, toasted,
   coarsely chopped

1 / Combine 2 tablespoons of the reserved orange juice and the olive oil in a small bowl.

2 / Spray a large frying pan with oil and heat on high. Season the kangaroo with pepper and cook it in the hot pan for 1–2 minutes each side until well browned but still medium-rare. Transfer to a plate lined with paper towel, and cover with foil to keep warm. (The paper towel soaks up the meat juices, ensuring they won't run into the salad.)

3 / On a large plate, arrange the witlof, rocket, mint and orange segments. Thickly slice the kangaroo and add to the plate. Drizzle the dressing over and sprinkle with hazelnuts.

TIPS / While kangaroo doesn't have any fat, be sure to trim off any sinew, as it can be chewy. / Make sure the pan is really hot before adding the kangaroo – it needs to be cooked rare or medium to remain tender. / Seedless oranges are easier to segment than the seed-filled kind.

VARIATION / You can also make this salad with 200 g of chicken breast (388 calories per serve) or with 250 g of pork fillet (389 calories per serve) instead of kangaroo.

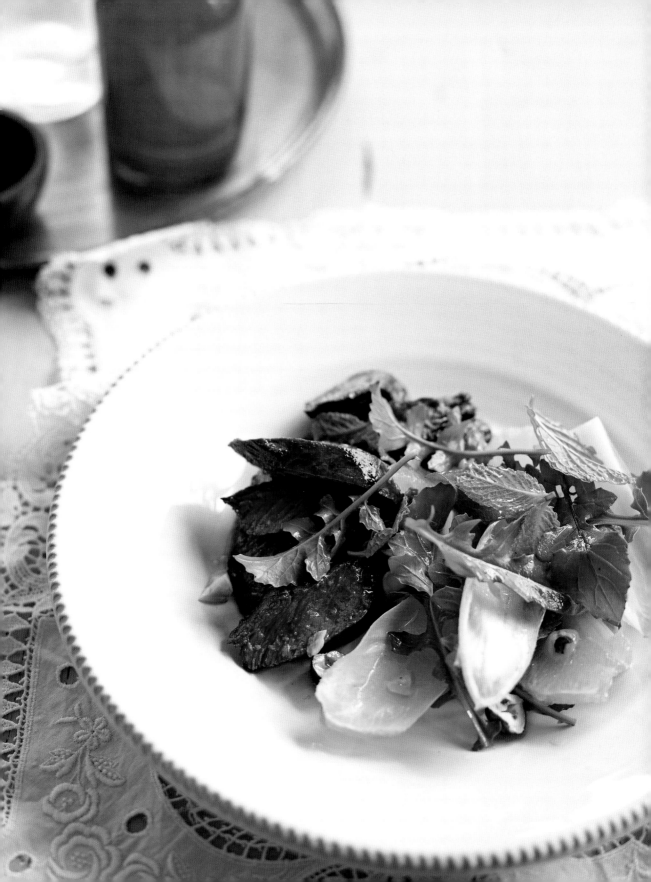

Kangaroo and tomato, basil and bocconcini skewers

What's the Italian for 'kangaroo'? This dish! It's another great way to introduce kangaroo into your diet, plus skewers tend to slow down the eating process, which gets a tick of approval from me.

SERVES 2 / *PREP* 15 mins / *COOK* 5 mins / *CAL PER SERVE* 380

250 g cherry tomatoes
1 cup basil leaves
150 g bocconcini, drained and halved
300 g kangaroo fillet, trimmed

and cut into 4 cm cubes
cracked black pepper
1 lemon wedge, thinly sliced
2 teaspoons extra virgin olive oil

1 | Heat the barbecue on high.

2 | Thread the tomatoes, basil and bocconcini alternately onto 10 small skewers.

3 | Season the kangaroo with pepper and thread it and the lemon slices onto 6 skewers, starting and finishing each skewer with a slice of lemon.

4 | Barbecue the kangaroo skewers for 2 minutes, turning regularly, until well browned but rare to medium inside.

5 | Serve the tomato skewers and kangaroo skewers together, drizzled with olive oil.

TIPS | If you're using wooden skewers, soak them in water for 30 minutes beforehand to avoid scorching them. | Make sure the barbecue is really hot before adding the kangaroo, and don't be tempted to cook it for longer than the stated cooking time, or it'll be tough. For the same reason, chop your kangaroo cubes no smaller than 4 cm, or they'll be overcooked inside before they're browned outside.

VARIATION | These skewers are also delicious made with 250 g of grass-fed beef fillet (401 calories per serve).

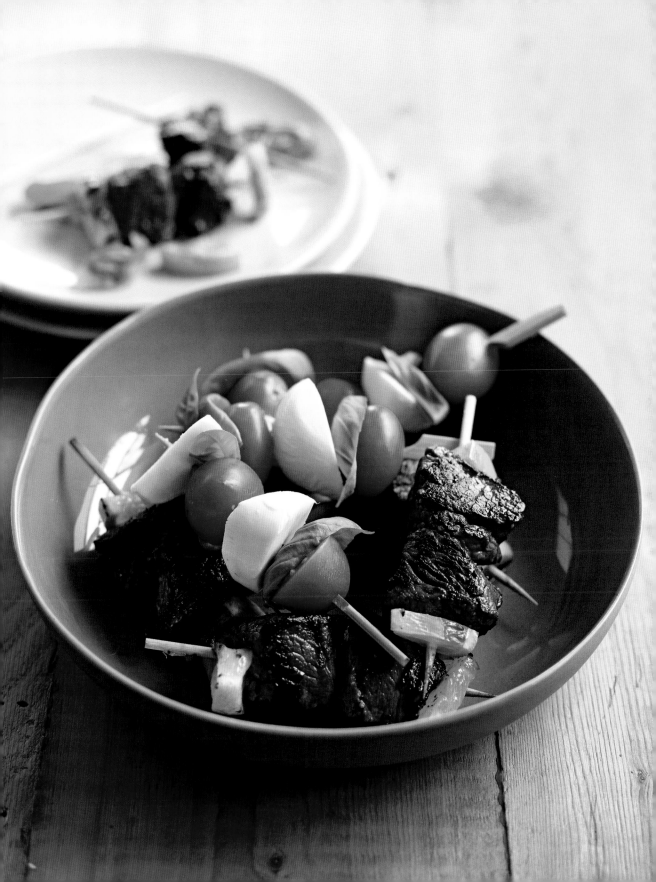

Grilled salmon with broccolini and pine nut salad

Any dish with both fish and greens and you've got me sitting up! The nutrients in this meal alone will blow your mind! You may just have to brace yourself for how amazing you'll feel after eating it.

SERVES 2 | *PREP* 10 mins | *COOK* 10 mins | *CAL PER SERVE* 406

olive oil spray

1 red onion, cut into wedges

2 × 150 g salmon fillets

cracked black pepper

2 bunches broccolini, trimmed

2 teaspoons lemon juice

1 teaspoon extra virgin olive oil

2 tablespoons pine nuts, toasted

lemon wedges, to serve

1 | Put a small saucepan of water on to boil.

2 | Lightly spray a char-grill pan with oil and heat it on medium–high. Add the onion and cook, turning occasionally, for 3 minutes, until softened and lightly charred. Remove and set aside.

3 | Spray the char-grill with more oil. Season the salmon with pepper, and cook on the grill for 5–6 minutes, turning once, until lightly charred and medium (the flesh should be opaque).

4 | Meanwhile, steam the broccolini over the boiling water for 5 minutes or until just tender. Combine the lemon juice and olive oil, then toss through the broccolini and onion in a bowl. Sprinkle with the pine nuts.

5 | Serve the salmon with lemon wedges and the broccolini salad alongside.

VARIATION | You can grill 2 × 150 g beef fillets instead of the salmon, if you're in the mood for red meat (385 calories per serve).

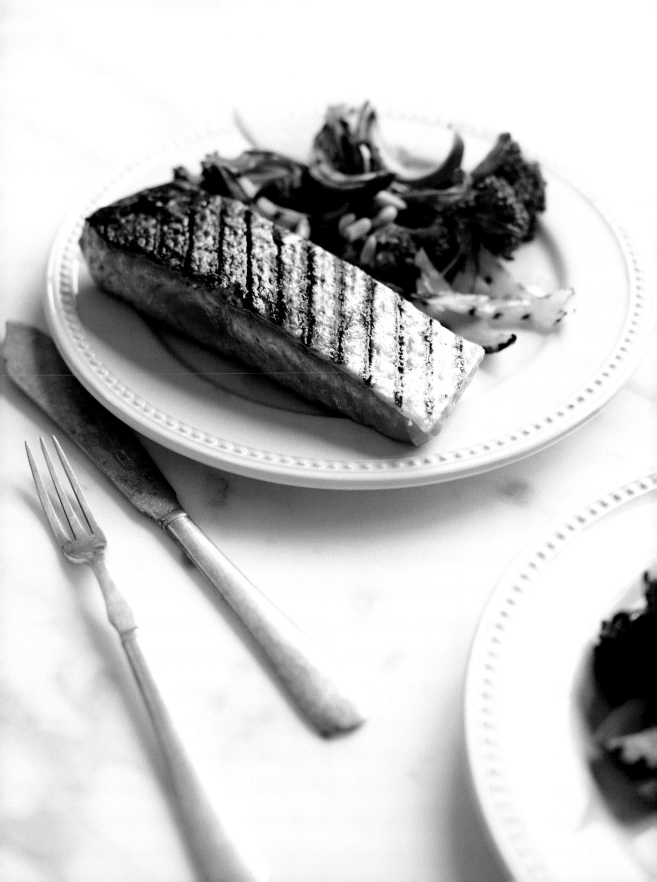

Portuguese octopus salad with giardiniera

Okay, I'm not trying to go all *MasterChef* on you here, but this is totally *yummo*! And dead easy! A beautiful summertime meal.

SERVES 2 | *PREP* 20 mins | *COOK* 20 mins | *CAL PER SERVE* 404

1 kg octopus, cleaned

salt

3 tomatoes, diced

1 small green capsicum, diced

½ onion, diced

150 g drained *giardiniera*, coarsely chopped, plus ¼ cup of *giardiniera* liquid

1 cup coarsely chopped fresh coriander

1 tablespoon extra virgin olive oil

cracked black pepper

1 | Place the octopus in a saucepan, cover with water and season with salt. Bring to the boil, then simmer, covered, for 20 minutes until just tender. Drain.

2 | When the octopus is cool enough to handle, discard the outer skin from the tentacles and thickly slice.

3 | Combine the octopus with the remaining ingredients in a large bowl. Season with pepper and toss to coat, then serve.

TIPS | Ask your fishmonger to clean the octopus for you. | You can cook and cool the octopus in advance, but don't toss the salad together until just before serving. | *Giardiniera* are pickled vegetables that are used in Portuguese, Italian and Greek cooking. They're sold in jars in delis and supermarkets. The mix of vegetables varies, but usually includes carrots, cauliflower, onion, gherkins and capsicum.

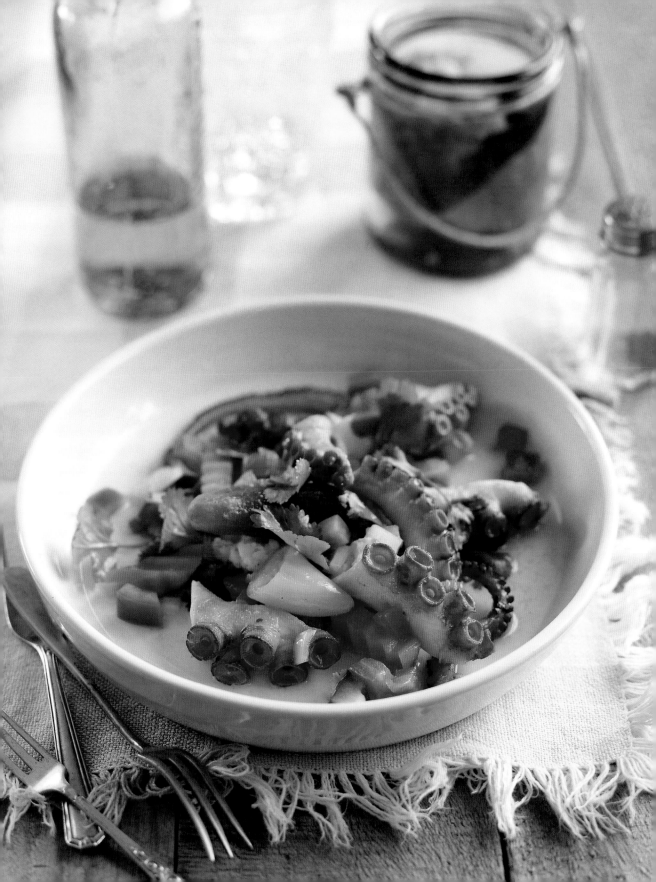

Spicy Moroccan patties

Big hit! These are easy and fun to make, so get the kids involved.
The patties are great in lunch boxes and taste just as good the next day.

SERVES 2 | *PREP* 30 mins | *COOK* 10 mins | *CAL PER SERVE* 356

1 teaspoon olive oil
4 cloves garlic, crushed
3 teaspoons ras el hanout
100 g stale wholemeal bread
400 g canned brown lentils,
    drained and rinsed
1 small egg
1 cup finely chopped mint

1 cup finely chopped parsley
cracked black pepper
2/3 cup low-cal yoghurt
harissa, to taste
2 tomatoes, sliced
½ red onion, thinly sliced
olive oil spray

1 / Heat the oil in a large non-stick frying pan on medium. Add the garlic and ras el hanout, and cook for 30 seconds until fragrant. Remove and set aside.

2 / Put the bread into a food processor and process it into breadcrumbs. Add the garlic mixture, lentils, egg, half the mint and half the parsley. Season with pepper and process until combined. With wet hands, shape the mixture into 10 patties.

3 / Combine the yoghurt, remaining herbs and a little harissa in a small bowl. Arrange the tomatoes and onion on a plate.

4 / Spray the frying pan with oil and heat on medium. Cook the patties for 4 minutes each side until browned. Serve with a dollop of yoghurt and the tomato and onion salad alongside.

TIPS | Ras el hanout is a wonderful Moroccan blend of spices. | Use the harissa sparingly – it's a very hot chilli paste! | You can keep the patty mixture in the fridge overnight and cook the patties the next day, if pressed for time.

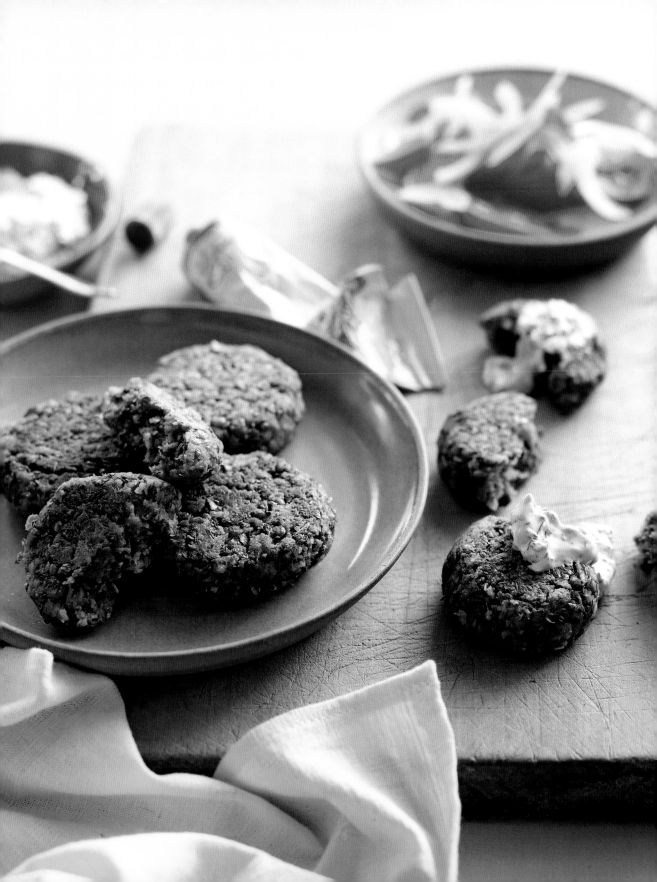

Perfect veggie casserole

This dish really gets me excited! Not only is it easy to put together, it will freeze well for future meals. It's super adaptable – you can add things like fish, chicken, beef or extra greens to it. And it's *really* good for you. *And* it tastes great! What more could you want? Cook it!

SERVES 6 | *PREP* 15 mins | *COOK* 1 hr 10 mins | *CAL PER SERVE* 304

3 medium eggplants, cut into chunks
2 teaspoons olive oil
1 onion, chopped
4 cloves garlic, thinly sliced
1 bay leaf
3 x 400 g cans chickpeas,
    drained and rinsed

2 x 400 g cans diced tomato
2 red capsicums, cut into chunks
2 medium zucchini, thickly sliced
100 g baby spinach
¾ cup pitted kalamata olives, drained,
    rinsed and thickly sliced
1 cup torn basil leaves

1 | Over a saucepan of simmering water, steam the eggplant for 6 minutes until just tender. Set aside.

2 | Meanwhile, heat the oil in a large heavy-based casserole dish on medium. Add the onion, garlic and bay leaf, and cook for 5 minutes, stirring, until softened. Add the chickpeas, tomato, capsicum, zucchini, drained eggplant and ½ cup of water. Stir until combined. Bring to the boil, then reduce the heat to low and cook, covered, for 1 hour until the vegetables are tender.

3 | Stir through the spinach, olives and basil, and serve.

TIP | Freeze single portions of this casserole in airtight containers.

VARIATION | Half a serve of veggie casserole goes beautifully with 150 g grilled chicken breast fillet (355 calories) or 150 g of lean lamb steak or fillet (369 calories)

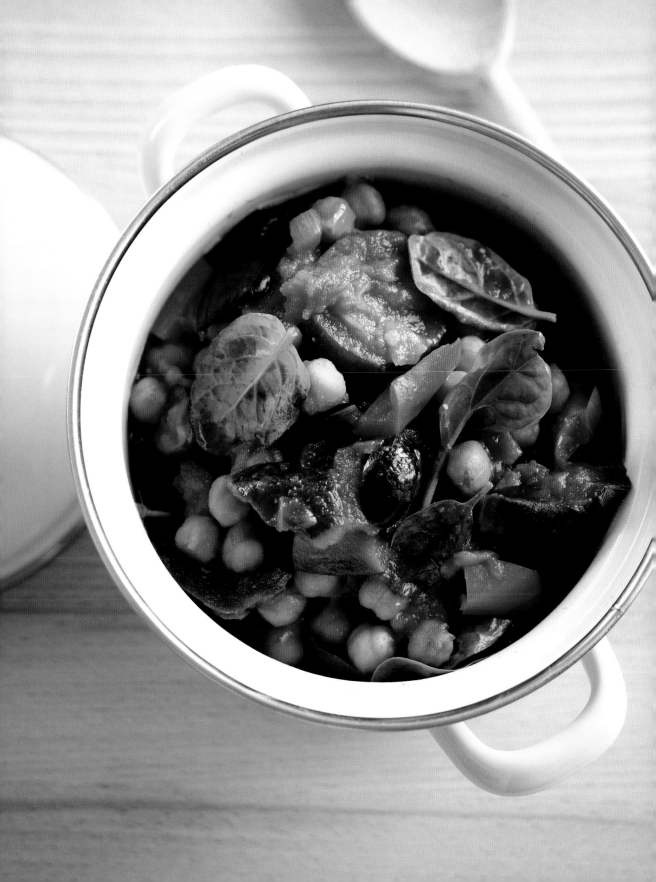

Tandoori veggies with raita

If you've had trouble getting your kids to eat veggies, this has got to be the way to go. I love the Indian vibe to this dish and the raita is just heavenly. One of those dishes that make you a kitchen rock star!

SERVES 2 | *PREP* 20 mins | *COOK* 45 mins | *CAL PER SERVE* 343

3 teaspoons garam masala
1 teaspoon ground turmeric
1 teaspoon cumin seeds
dried chilli flakes, to taste
1 turnip, peeled and quartered
2 carrots, quartered lengthways
2 zucchini, cut into chunks
1 onion, halved
400 g pumpkin, cut into wedges
2 teaspoons vegetable oil

Raita
1 Lebanese cucumber
salt
1 cup low-cal yoghurt
½ cup finely chopped mint
½ clove garlic, crushed

1 | Preheat the oven to 220°C/200°C fan-forced.

2 | Combine all the spices in a small bowl. Put the vegetables into a large roasting tray, then add the oil and the spice mix. Rub the oil and spice mix over the veggies with your hands to coat them well. Roast for 45 minutes or until tender.

3 | While the veggies are roasting, make the raita. Coarsely grate the cucumber, tip it into a fine sieve, season it with salt and let it stand over a bowl for 15 minutes. This will draw out some of the moisture in the cucumber, so it's not too wet. Rinse the cucumber under cold water and drain well, squeezing out all the moisture, then combine it with the other raita ingredients in a bowl. Refrigerate until you're ready to serve.

4 | Serve the roasted vegetables with the raita alongside.

TIP | If you're pressed for time, you could use a ready-made tandoori spice mix from your local supermarket instead.

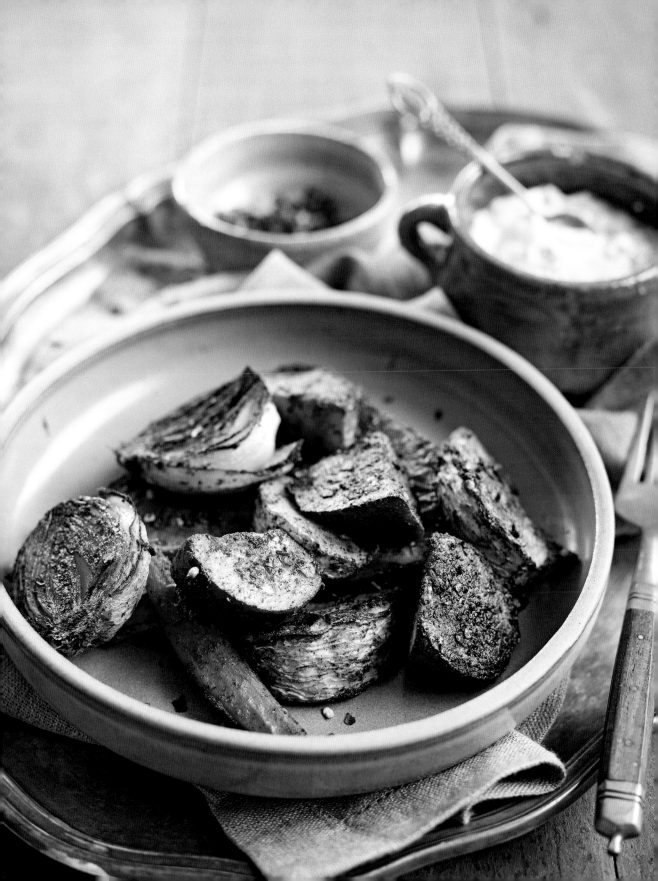

Chicken stir-fry with brussels sprouts and almonds

Brussels sprouts are just bursting with nutrients; you would be bonkers not to eat them. I love their flavour mixed with almonds too. This is a really nice take on a stir-fry.

SERVES 2 | *PREP* 15 mins | *COOK* 15 mins | *CAL PER SERVE* 325

2 tablespoons slivered almonds
cooking oil spray
1 red capsicum, thinly sliced
200 g skinless chicken breast, thinly sliced

400 g brussels sprouts, trimmed and halved
3 cloves garlic, thinly sliced
1 tablespoon hoisin sauce
2 teaspoons low-salt soy sauce

1 | Heat a wok on medium. Stir-fry the almonds until toasted, then set aside.

2 | Lightly spray the wok with oil. Stir-fry the capsicum for 2 minutes, until lightly charred and just tender. Set aside.

3 | Lightly spray the wok with oil again. Stir-fry the chicken for 2 minutes until browned and cooked. Set aside. Stir-fry the brussels sprouts and garlic for 3 minutes until golden. Add ¾ cup of water and simmer the sprouts for 6 minutes, loosely covered with a saucepan lid, until just tender and the water has evaporated.

4 | Return the chicken to the pan along with the capsicum and sauces, and stir-fry until everything is well coated with sauce and heated through.

5 | Serve the stir-fry sprinkled with the toasted almonds.

VARIATION | Trimmed and sliced steak (250 g) makes a nice change from the chicken and has about the same calories (350 calories per serve). Just make sure you don't overcook the beef, or it'll be tough.

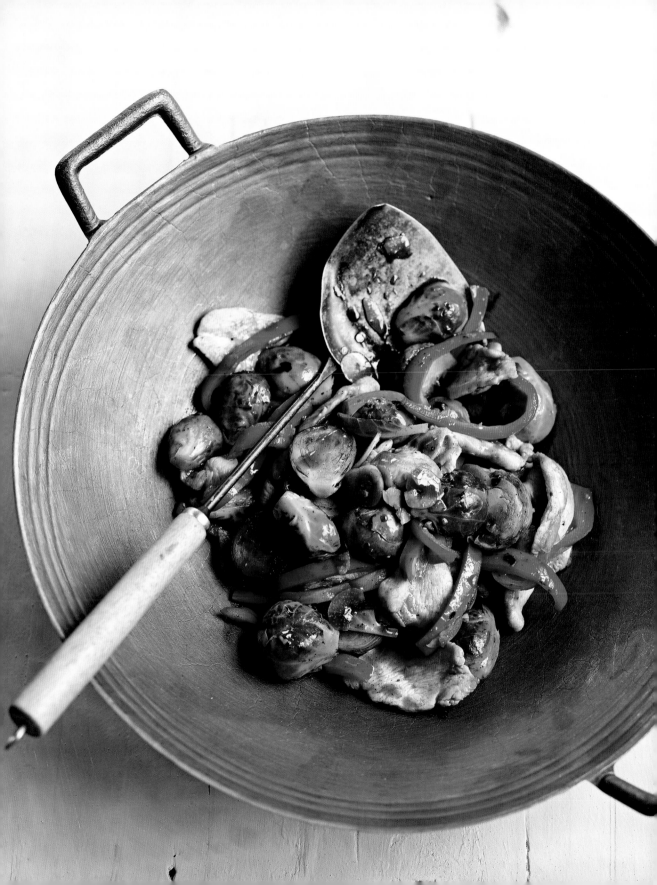

Lamb fillet with spinach, red cabbage and mint salad

Hello? Lamb and mint! That's got to be one of the most heavenly flavour combinations ever! And then add spinach to that? This dish could be the 'holy grail' of superfoods! Last supper, anyone?

SERVES 2 | *PREP* 20 mins | *COOK* 10 mins | *CAL PER SERVE* 340

¼ cup low-cal yoghurt
1 cup mint leaves
1 bunch asparagus, trimmed
250 g lamb fillet, trimmed
cracked black pepper

150 g red cabbage, shredded
75 g baby spinach
2 tablespoons macadamia nuts, coarsely chopped

1 | Put a small saucepan of salted water on to boil.

2 | Meanwhile, to make the dressing, process the yoghurt and half the mint in a food processor until smooth.

3 | Add the asparagus to the boiling water, and cook for 2 minutes until just tender. Meanwhile, crack some ice into a bowl of cold water. When the asparagus is done, drain and tip it into the iced water. Then drain again and cut into chunks.

4 | Lightly spray a frying pan with oil and heat on high. Season the lamb fillet with pepper, and cook it for 2 minutes each side until well browned but medium on the inside. Set aside, loosely covered with foil, for 2 minutes to rest, before slicing it thickly.

5 | Combine the cabbage, spinach, asparagus and the remaining mint in a bowl, then add the lamb and toss.

6 | Arrange the salad on two plates, drizzle with the dressing and sprinkle the macadamia nuts over.

TIP | You can also use 300 g of pork fillet instead of the lamb (323 calories per serve).

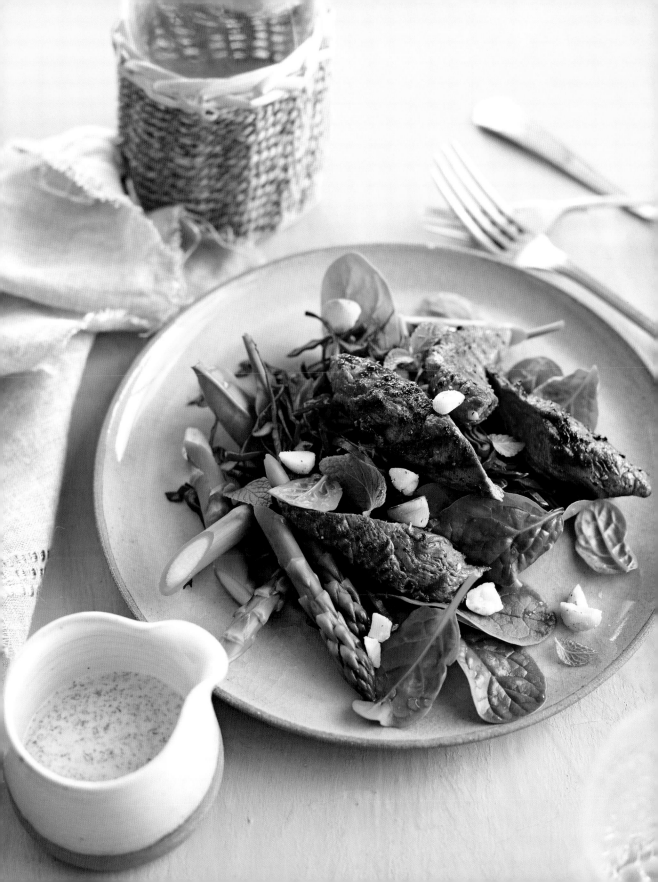

Capsicums stuffed with beef and zucchini

I love a nice stuffed capsicum myself! And this one totally rocks. Super tasty, and it looks really special on the plate. A brilliant way to get your veggie on!

SERVES 2 / *PREP* 10 mins / *COOK* 45 mins / *CAL PER SERVE* 339

180 g lean beef mince

1 large zucchini, coarsely grated

¼ cup couscous

2 tablespoons chopped parsley

2 tablespoons grated parmesan cheese

2 spring onions, finely chopped

2 large red capsicums

50 g mixed salad leaves

1 / Preheat the oven to 220°C/200°C fan-forced.

2 / Combine the beef, zucchini, couscous, parsley, parmesan and onion in a medium bowl.

3 / Slice the tops off the capsicums. Discard the seeds and membranes. Spoon the beef mixture into the capsicums and replace the tops. Wrap each capsicum in foil and roast for 30 minutes.

4 / Open the foil – being careful not to burn yourself! – and roast the capsicums for another 15 minutes.

5 / Serve with the mixed leaves alongside.

TIP / It's important to choose capsicums that will stand upright in your oven, or things could get very messy!

VARIATIONS / Chicken mince (344 calories per serve) or lean lamb mince (339 calories per serve) are also great instead of the beef, and spices such as curry powder or a Moroccan spice mix add even more flavour to the stuffing.

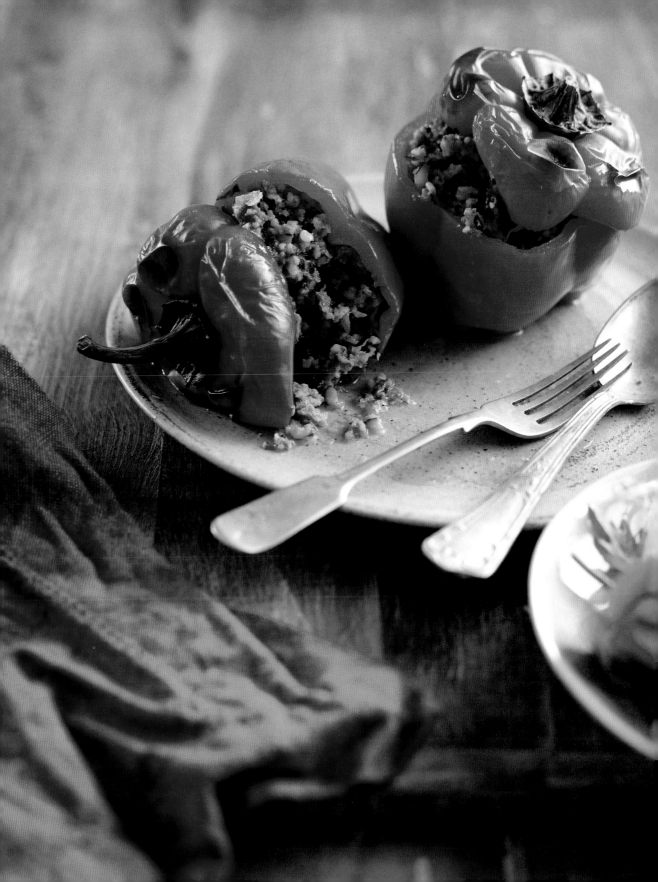

Grilled liver with garlic broccoli and cherry tomatoes

Okay, hear me out! I would not put liver in a recipe if it wasn't 'ruler supreme' when it comes to nutrients. I know what you're thinking: 'How will I get my kids/husband/wife/new boyfriend to eat this?' Simple. Don't tell them. Bask in the glory that you are extending their life by serving a truly *super* food.

SERVES 2 | *PREP* 15 mins | *COOK* 10 mins | *CAL PER SERVE* 316

finely grated zest of 1 lemon

2 tablespoons chopped parsley

1 teaspoon olive oil

250 g cherry tomatoes, halved

3 cloves garlic, thinly sliced

400 g broccoli, trimmed and broken into florets

2 teaspoons lemon juice

olive oil spray

250 g calves' liver

1 | Combine the lemon zest and parsley in a small bowl, then set aside.

2 | Heat the oil in a wok on high. Stir-fry the tomatoes and garlic for 2 minutes until the tomatoes are lightly charred and the garlic is golden. Set aside.

3 | Stir-fry the broccoli for 2 minutes until lightly charred, add ⅓ cup of water to the wok, and cook, loosely covered with a saucepan lid, for 3 minutes until the broccoli is just tender and the water has evaporated. Return the tomatoes and garlic to the wok and stir-fry until hot, then drizzle the lemon juice over.

4 | Meanwhile, lightly spray a frying pan with olive oil and heat it on high. Add the liver and cook for 2 minutes (if thickly cut) or until well browned and cooked to your liking.

5 | Serve the liver sprinkled with the parsley mixture alongside the stir-fried broccoli and tomatoes.

TIP | Don't overcook the liver or it will be tough. If your pieces are thin, they won't need as much cooking time – keep an eye on them. The liver is cooked when it is firm but springy to the touch. Alternatively, cut through the liver; it should be slightly pink inside.

VARIATION | The liver has a wonderful flavour, but this recipe is also great with 350 g of trimmed, grass-fed steak instead (338 calories per serve).

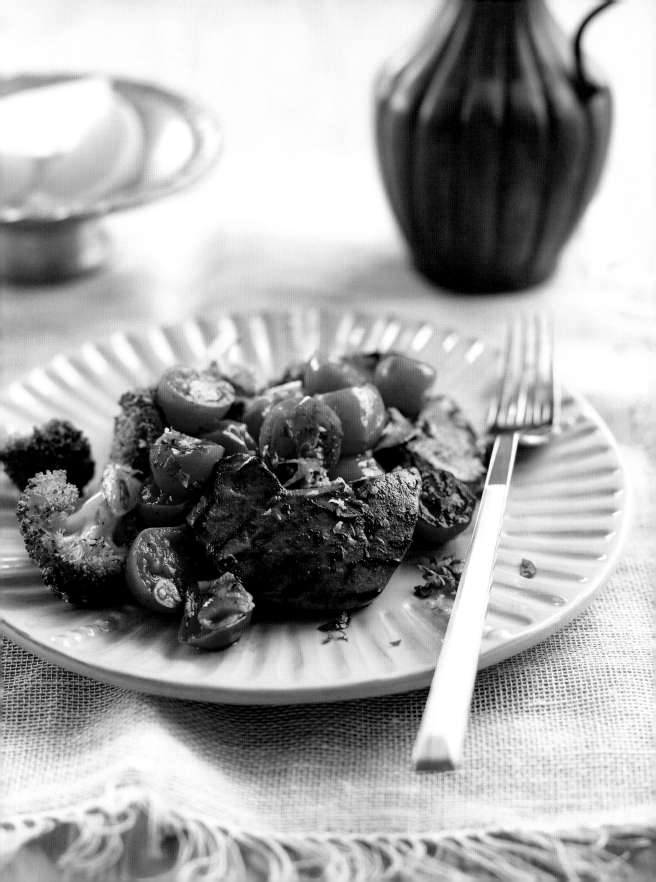

Steak and green beans with warm tomato and basil dressing

This is a good old meat and veg dish with a zingy twist in the dressing. Simple. Tasty. Nutritious. It's a total winner!

SERVES 2 / *PREP* 15 mins / *COOK* 10 mins / *CAL PER SERVE* 327

200 g green beans, trimmed
200 g butter beans, trimmed
olive oil spray
350 g rump steak, trimmed
cracked black pepper
2 teaspoons extra virgin olive oil

2 cloves garlic, crushed
4 anchovy fillets, drained and
  finely chopped
2 Roma tomatoes, diced
½ cup torn basil leaves

1 / Bring a medium-sized saucepan of salted water to the boil. Add the beans and bring back to the boil. Cook for 4–5 minutes until tender, then drain the beans and return them to the pan. Cover to keep them warm.

2 / Meanwhile, lightly spray a frying pan with oil and heat on high. Season the steaks with pepper and cook for 1 minute each side for rare, or until cooked to your liking. Set aside, loosely covered with foil, to keep warm.

3 / In the frying pan, heat the oil on medium and cook the garlic and anchovy for 1 minute until fragrant. Add the tomato and cook, stirring, until it starts to soften. Stir in the basil, remove from the heat and season with pepper.

4 / Plate up the steaks and the beans, then spoon the tomato mixture over the top.

VARIATION / You could also pan-fry 2 × 200 g white fish fillets instead of the beef (338 calories per serve), if you're in the mood for something lighter.

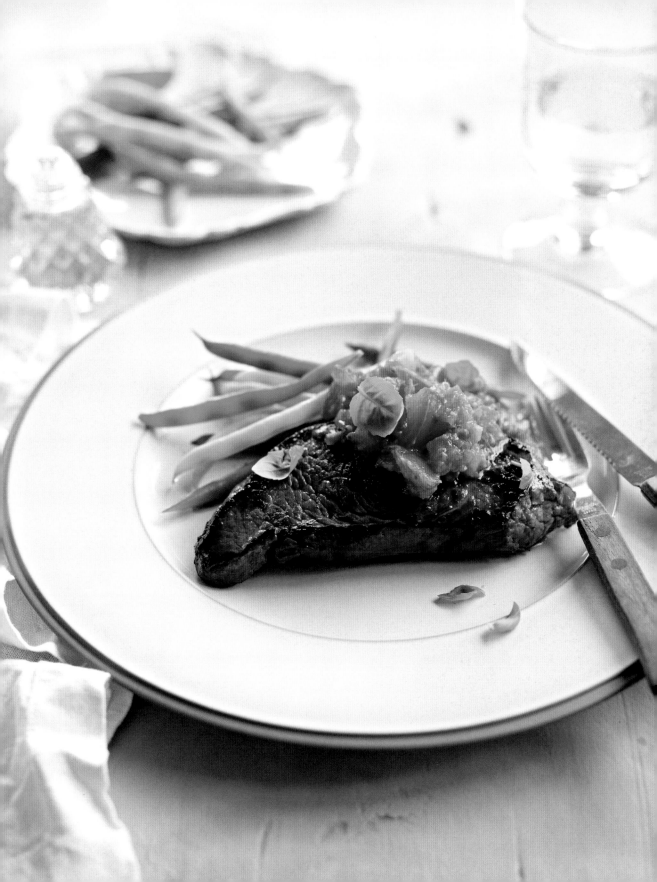

Beef and silverbeet stir-fry

I haven't come across anyone who doesn't like this dish, and I have to say it is jammed with nutrients. Silverbeet is a total star when it comes to superfoods, and this dish is just so easy to put together.

SERVES 2 | *PREP* 20 mins | *COOK* 15 mins | *CAL PER SERVE* 339

1 bunch silverbeet, trimmed
cooking oil spray
1 bunch asparagus, trimmed,
   cut into chunks
100 g baby corn, halved lengthways
1 large carrot, thinly sliced on the diagonal

4 cm piece fresh ginger, peeled
   and cut into matchsticks
300 g rump steak, trimmed and
   thinly sliced
2 tablespoons oyster sauce
1 tablespoon low-salt soy sauce

1 | Thinly slice the stems of the silverbeet and set aside. Cut away and discard the white centre vein from the leaves, and coarsely shred the green part of the leaves.

2 | Lightly spray a large wok with oil and heat on medium–high. Stir-fry the asparagus, corn, carrot and ginger for 6 minutes until just tender. Add the silverbeet stems and stir-fry for 3 minutes. Tip the vegetables into a bowl.

3 | Lightly spray the wok with oil again and increase the heat to high. Stir-fry the beef in two batches for about 1 minute, until browned but still rare inside. Add the silverbeet leaves and stir-fry until wilted.

4 | Return the vegetables to the wok, as well as the sauces. Stir-fry until well coated and hot. Serve immediately.

TIPS | This may seem like a huge amount of silverbeet leaves, but it wilts down to nothing. If you don't have a wok big enough to fit it all in one go, stir-fry it in batches. | Make sure you only just brown the beef, or it will overcook and be tough – it continues to cook when it's stirred through at the end.

VARIATION | Kale can be used instead of silverbeet if you want even more nutrients!

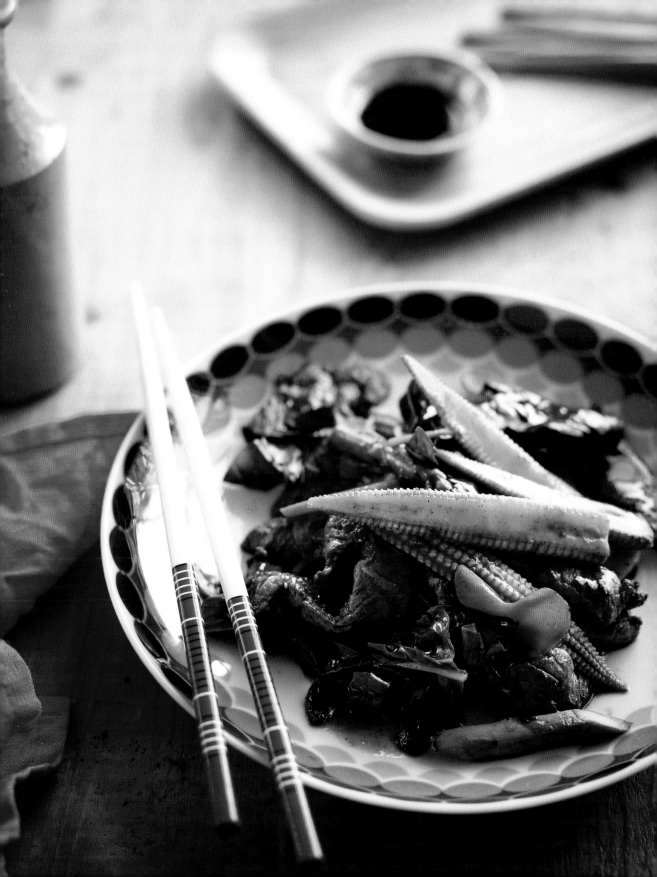

Poached blue-eye with spinach and grapefruit salad

Divine! That's really all I can say about this dish! Cook it. Eat it. Love it!

SERVES 2 | **PREP** 20 mins | **COOK** 10 mins | **CAL PER SERVE** 332

200 g snow peas, trimmed
1 bunch asparagus, trimmed
  and cut into chunks
400 g blue-eye trevalla fillets

100 g baby spinach
100 g radish, cut into batons
1 yellow grapefruit, segmented
1 tablespoon extra virgin olive oil

1 | Bring a small saucepan of salted water to the boil. Add the snow peas and asparagus. Boil for 2 minutes. Cool in iced water. Drain well.

2 | Place the blue-eye in a large saucepan and just cover with water. Bring to a gentle simmer. Remove from the heat. Allow to stand, covered, for 3 minutes. Remove the fish with a slotted egg flip.

3 | Meanwhile, combine the snow peas, asparagus, spinach, radish and grapefruit in a bowl. Drizzle with oil and toss to combine.

4 | Serve the fish with the salad alongside.

TIPS | Choose a seedless grapefruit. | Poaching is great as it makes it hard to overcook the fish, but you can also char-grill or pan-fry the fish fillets. The cooking time will vary depending on the thickness of the fillet. The fish should easily flake with a fork when done.

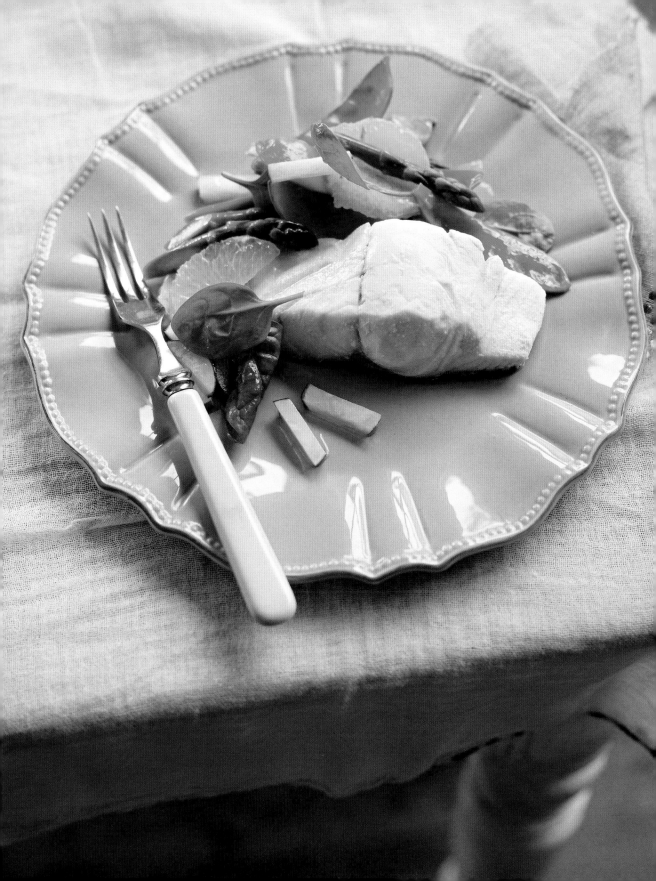

Chinese steamed whole whiting

Now this dish is a statement! Every time I have put this on the table it's been greeted with 'oohs' and 'aahs' all round. It's great for the body, but the compliments are also great for the soul!

SERVES 2 / *PREP* 20 mins / *COOK* 15 mins / *CAL PER SERVE* 360

4 cm piece fresh ginger,
   peeled and cut into batons
2 x 350 g whole whiting,
   gutted and scaled
1 large carrot, cut into batons
1 large zucchini, cut into batons

100 g shiitake mushrooms, sliced
200 g snow peas, thinly sliced
2 teaspoons low-sodium soy sauce
1 teaspoon sesame oil
¼ cup coriander sprigs
1 spring onion, trimmed, shredded

1 / Put a steamer saucepan on to simmer.

2 / Scatter half of the ginger in a steamer basket large enough to fit both fish in a single layer. Put the remaining ginger inside the cavity of each fish and place the whiting in the basket. Place the steamer basket over the saucepan of simmering water. Steam for 10–15 minutes, until the flesh is opaque and comes easily away from the backbone.

3 / Meanwhile, place the carrot, zucchini, mushrooms and snow peas in a second steamer basket. Steam for 5 minutes.

4 / Reserve a spoonful of the vegetables. Divide the remaining vegetables between two large plates. Top with the fish. Combine the soy sauce and oil, and drizzle over the fish. Scatter the reserved vegetables, coriander and onion over.

TIP / Use Chinese bamboo steam baskets that you can stack.

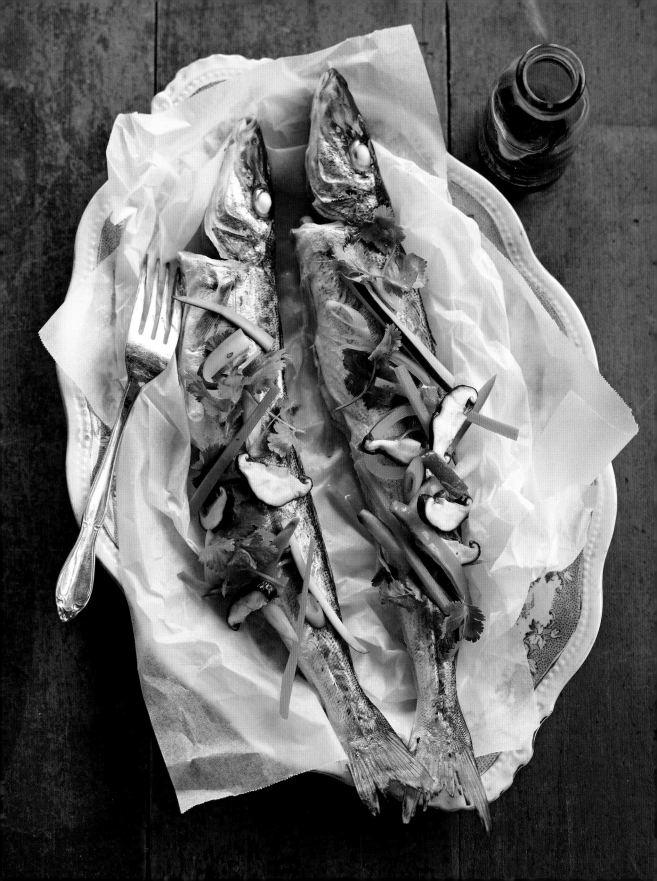

Red prawn curry

Who says that curries have to be off the menu when you are looking to stay slim and fighting fit? Well not me, not with this dish. Everyone loves a curry and now you can enjoy one in a healthy, tasty way!

SERVES 2 / *PREP* 25 mins / *COOK* 10 mins / *CAL PER SERVE* 362

1 tablespoon red curry paste

1¼ cups light coconut-flavoured
   evaporated milk

1 bunch asparagus, trimmed and
   cut into chunks

200 g green beans, trimmed and halved

1 large zucchini, thinly sliced

50 g baby corn, halved

400 g medium green prawns,
   peeled and deveined, tails left on

1 teaspoon fish sauce

½ cup Thai basil leaves

1 / Heat the curry paste in a medium-sized saucepan on medium heat for 30 seconds until fragrant. Stir in the evaporated milk. Add the asparagus, beans, zucchini and corn. Gently simmer, without boiling, for 5 minutes until just tender. Remove the vegetables from the pan with a slotted spoon and set aside. Cover to keep warm.

2 / Add the prawns and fish sauce to the saucepan. Gently simmer, without boiling, for about 4 minutes, until the prawns are pink and opaque. Return the vegetables to the pan along with half the basil and cook until hot.

3 / Serve scattered with the remaining basil leaves.

TIPS / You can also leave the heads on the prawns, if desired. Some consider them the most flavoursome part. / Do not bring the curry to the boil or it may split. / Use ordinary basil if you can't find any Thai basil.

VARIATION / You can use 200 g thinly sliced chicken breast fillet instead of the prawns (391 calories per serve).

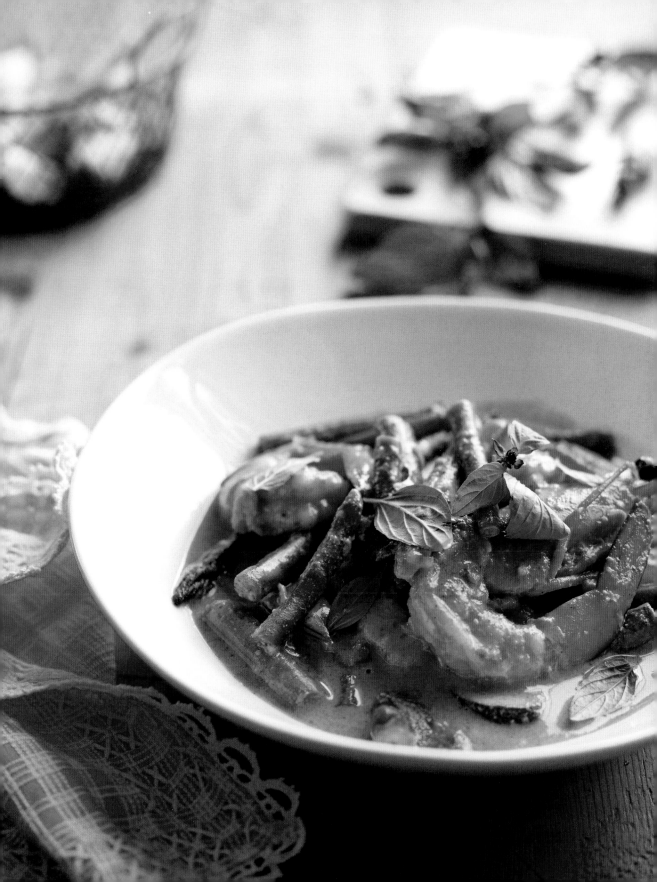

Billy's prawn cocktail salad

My husband, Billy, came up with this dish one Christmas time and its been the talk of the town ever since! You can serve it in martini glasses for a touch of Art Deco glamour. Go on, I dare you!

SERVES 2 | *PREP* 25 mins | *COOK* 5 mins | *CAL PER SERVE* 319

100 g green beans, trimmed
100 g snow peas, trimmed
100 g sugar snap peas, trimmed
¼ cup low-cal yoghurt
1 teaspoon lemon juice

1 teaspoon Dijon mustard
400 g cooked medium prawns
250 g witlof, leaves separated
½ medium avocado, cut into wedges

1 | Bring a saucepan of salted water to the boil. Add the beans. Bring back to the boil and cook for 2 minutes. Add the snow peas and sugar snap peas. Cook for 2 minutes until just tender. Drain and cool in iced water. Drain again.

2 | To make the dressing, combine the yoghurt, lemon juice and mustard in a small bowl.

3 | Arrange the prawns, witlof, avocado and green vegetables on a large plate or in two martini glasses. Top with a dollop of the dressing.

TIP | Cook your own prawns. It's cheaper, they'll usually taste better, and you'll end up with a great stock for a fish soup. Simply boil the whole prawns in a small saucepan of salted water until pink and opaque. Drain, reserving the cooking liquid, and peel and devein when cooled. If you don't plan on eating the heads, return them to the pan with the cooking liquid and simmer for 30 minutes to intensify the flavour of the stock.

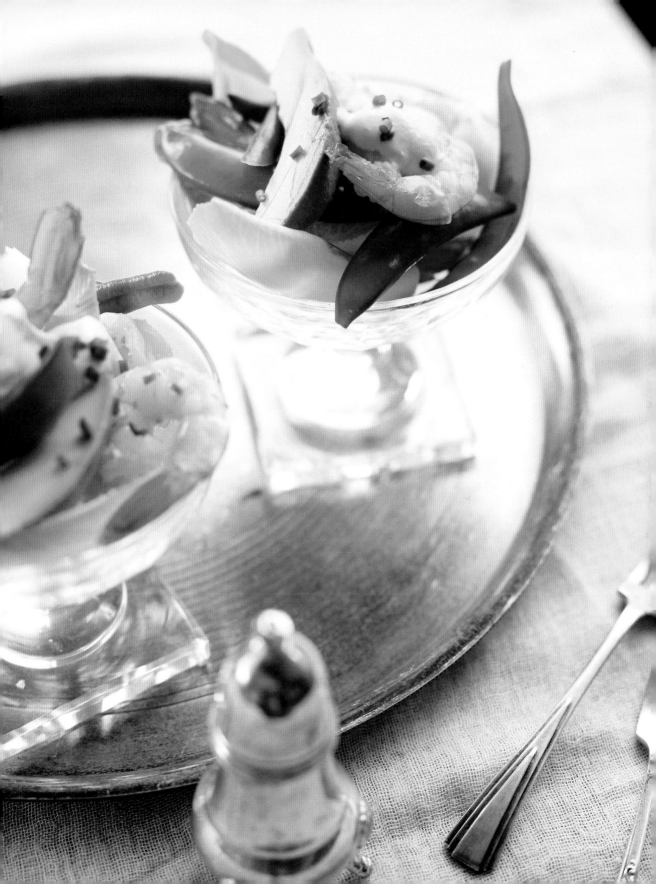

Mussels with tomato, onion and thyme

What a great meal this is. And the smell will transport you straight to Tuscany! I love the warm cosiness of this dish and the fact that cooking mussels this way tends to slow down the eating process. I must admit that a small glass of red wine does go well with this one.

SERVES 2 | *PREP* 20 mins | *COOK* 10 mins | *CAL PER SERVE* 359

1 kg mussels

1 teaspoon olive oil

1 onion, chopped

1 clove garlic, sliced

4 sprigs fresh thyme

½ long fresh red chilli, finely chopped

⅓ cup dry white wine

1 large tomato, diced

2 slices wholegrain bread

1 | Scrub the mussels under cold water and remove the beards. Discard any mussels that are cracked or that don't shut when you tap them.

2 | Heat the olive oil in a large saucepan on medium. Cook the onion, garlic, thyme and chilli for 5 minutes until softened. Increase the heat to high, then add the mussels and the wine. Cover and cook for 4 minutes or until the mussels open, stirring halfway through. Stir in the tomato until heated through.

3 | Meanwhile, toast the bread.

4 | Serve the mussels immediately in shallow bowls, with their cooking liquid spooned over and the toast on the side.

TIP | You can find ready-scrubbed bags of mussels at the fishmonger.

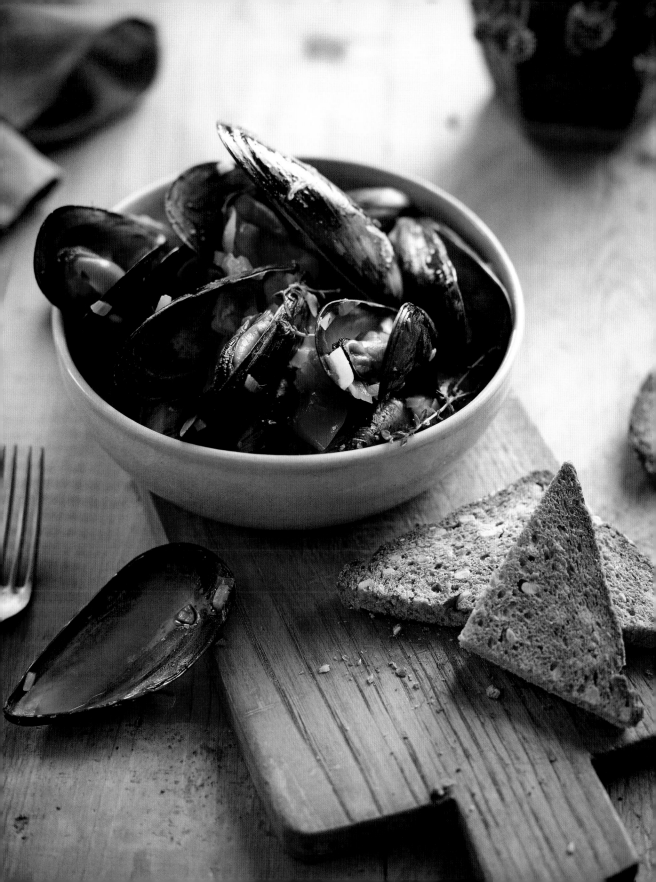

Raspberry rough

Raspberries are pumping with both antioxidants and fibre. So besides tasting sweet and decadent, you can be guaranteed you are totally looking after yourself with this dessert.

SERVES 4 / *PREP* 15 mins / *COOK* 5 mins / *CAL PER SERVE* 158

2 sheets filo pastry

cooking oil spray

200 g fresh raspberries

2 cups low-cal vanilla yoghurt

1 | Preheat the oven to 220°C/200°C fan-forced. Line an oven tray with baking paper.

2 | Lay one sheet of filo on a clean board and lightly spray with oil. Cover with the second sheet of filo and lightly spray with oil. Roll the pastry up tightly and cut into 2 cm logs with scissors. Unroll the logs into ribbons and place onto the prepared tray in eight small piles. Bake for 4–5 minutes until golden and crisp. Allow to cool on the tray.

3 | Spoon an eighth of the yoghurt into each of 4 glasses. Top with a few raspberries. Cover with an eighth of the filo. Then repeat to form a second layer of each ingredient. Serve immediately.

TIPS / You can make the filo strips up to 4 hours in advance. Store the cooled filo in an airtight container. / Assemble the dessert just before serving or the filo pastry will go soggy. / Store the remaining sheets of pastry in the refrigerator, wrapped in plastic wrap. You can also freeze filo. If doing so, freeze smaller batches wrapped in cling film.

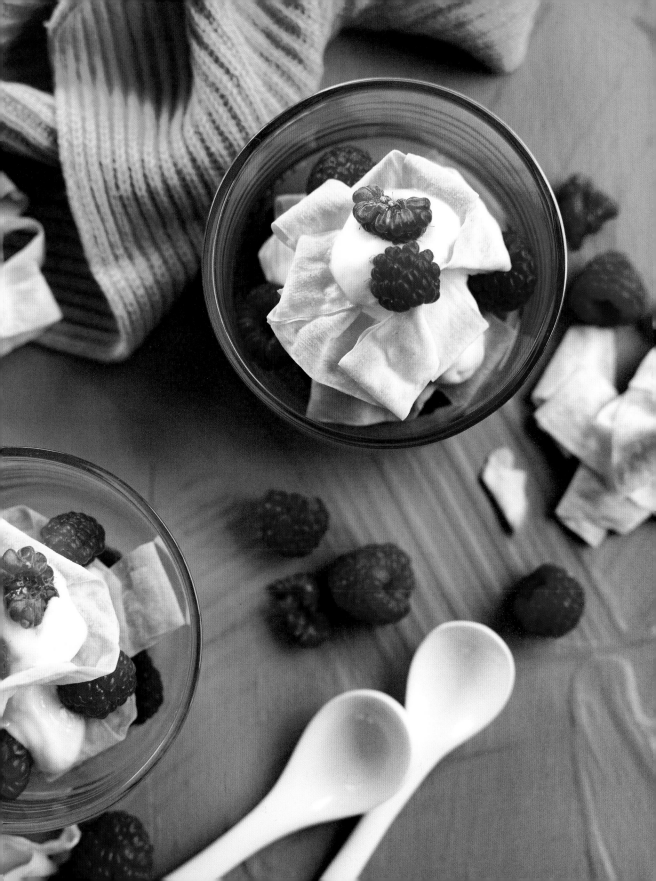

Very berry baked ricotta

OMG! This is divine! And it's good for you! I know. You can thank me later.

SERVES 2 / *PREP* 15 mins / *COOK* 25 mins / *CAL PER SERVE* 150

1⅓ cups low-cal ricotta cheese
1 small egg

150 g blueberries
250 g strawberries, hulled

1 / Preheat the oven to 200°C/180°C fan-forced. Lightly spray 4 holes of a muffin tray (⅓ cup-capacity).

2 / Whisk the ricotta and egg together in a small bowl until smooth. Stir through 50 g of the blueberries. Divide the mixture between 4 muffin holes and bake for 25 minutes until puffed, set and lightly golden. Allow to cool in the pan.

3 / Meanwhile, process 100 g of the strawberries in a small processor until smooth. Cut the remaining strawberries into quarters or halves depending on size.

4 / Place each baked ricotta onto a separate dessert plate, top with the remaining berries and drizzle with the strawberry purée.

TIPS / You can serve the baked ricotta slightly warm or at room temperature. / Choose ripe fruit as the sweetness of this dessert depends solely on the berries.

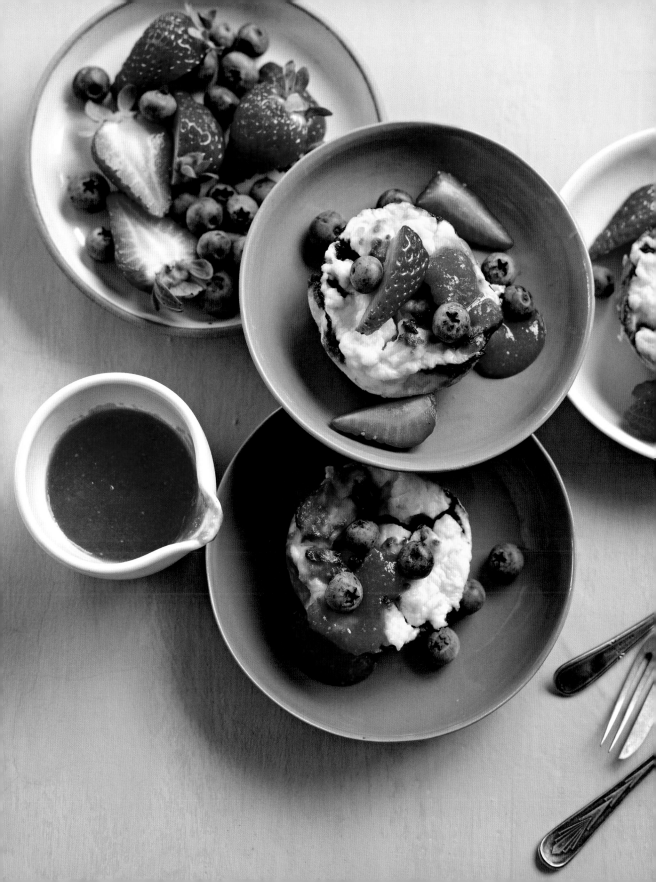

Strawberry yoghurt and kiwi popsicles

Really fun and really healthy! And you can rest assured that you are getting a goodly dose of vitamins in this one.

SERVES 4 | *PREP* 10 mins | *FREEZE* overnight | *CAL PER SERVE* 83

¾ cup low-cal vanilla yoghurt
250 g strawberries, hulled

3 kiwifruit, peeled and cored

1 | Process the yoghurt and strawberries together until smooth. Pour into four popsicle moulds, filling each about two-thirds full. Freeze for about 2 hours or until firm.

2 | Process the kiwifruit until smooth. Pour over the strawberry mixture. Insert a popsicle stick into each and freeze overnight until set.

TIP | Choose fruit that is nice and ripe. This will make your popsicles all the sweeter.

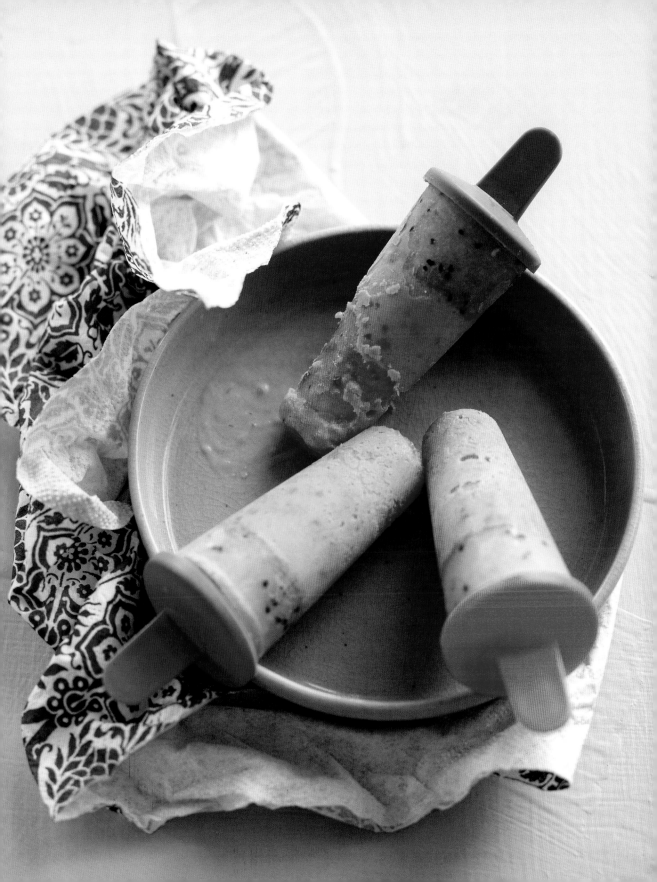

Baked apples

There's definitely something special about the smell of baked apples. It's homely, cosy and seriously mouth-watering! This dessert is a total winner with everyone.

SERVES 4 | *PREP* 10 mins | *COOK* 55 mins | *CAL PER SERVE* 151

¼ cup sultanas, finely chopped
2 tablespoons slivered almonds
1½ tablespoons rolled oats

1 teaspoon finely grated orange zest
4 medium apples

1 | Preheat the oven to 200°C /180°C fan-forced.

2 | Combine the sultanas, almonds, oats and orange rind in a small bowl.

3 | Slice the top off each apple and set the tops aside. Use a sharp knife or melon baller to remove the cores from the apples, leaving the apples whole and the bases intact. Spoon the sultana mixture into the centre of the apples. Replace the tops. Line a small metal roasting pan with foil, leaving enough each side to fold over the apples. Place the apples upright on the pan and fold the foil over the top. Bake for 45 minutes. Open the foil and bake for another 10 minutes.

4 | Serve warm.

TIP | A metal roasting pan is ideal for cooking the apples as it conducts the heat very efficiently. However, you can also use a ceramic dish; you will just need to cook the apples for a little longer.

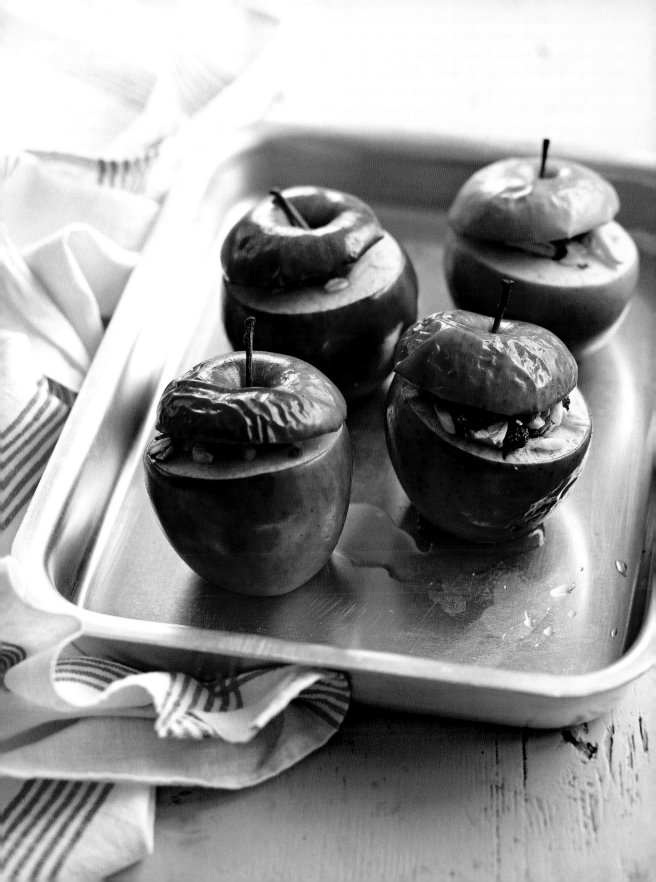

ACKNOWLEDGEMENTS

Putting a book like this together can only happen with the help and support of special people.

I owe a big thank you to Cindy and Jayne for sharing their lives with my readers, and to my 12 Week Body Transformation partners, Amelia and Tim, for helping me find them.

Thanks to Paul and Michael from Camperdown Fitness for providing me with an 'office' where I could develop my exercises as well as my body, and to my amazing personal trainer, Joey.

Morrie and Wally deserve my gratitude for not only letting me use their Balmain greengrocers for photographs, but also for providing me with wonderful fresh fruit and vegetables day after day.

To my dear friend Derek Hill from Life Fitness for the loan of his warehouse as well as his top-of-the-range gym equipment – thank you, you are a darling. And to my 'bestie', life coach Craig for his insights and for enhancing the photos in these pages with his amazing physique.

My gratitude to Nick Wilson for his flattering images, Alison Boyle for looking after my hair and makeup, and to 'the Penguins' – publisher Andrea McNamara, editor Daniel Hudspith, designer Adam Laszczuk, and the gorgeous Kirsten Abbott for her unswerving faith in me.

And of course my husband, Billy. His endless belief in me, and his support and wisdom, enabled me to get this book into your hands today.

INDEX